Endomorph Diet for Beginners

1000 Days of Balanced and Metabolism-Boosting Recipes with a 28-Day Meal Plan to Optimize Your Endomorph Nutrition | Full Color Edition

William D. Boyce

Editor: Aaliyah Lyons
Cover Art: Danielle Rees
Interior Design: Anilkumar N S
Food stylist: Sienna Adams

Contents

Introduction

In an era where fad diets and fleeting trends dominate the health and fitness landscape, it's refreshing to encounter an approach that prioritizes individuality and sustainable lifestyle changes. The Endomorph Diet recognizes that every person's body is distinctive, and as such, their nutritional requirements should be too. This cookbook stands as a beacon of evidence-based, practical wisdom, offering a pathway for endomorphs to achieve their health goals while celebrating the joy of food.

The journey to optimal well-being is not just about shedding pounds; it's about fostering a harmonious relationship between body, mind, and soul. The Endomorph Diet embraces this philosophy, promoting a holistic understanding of health that goes beyond mere aesthetics. As you embark on this adventure, remember that each recipe has been meticulously crafted to strike a balance between flavor and nutrition, ensuring that your taste buds dance with delight while your body thrives.

One of the most remarkable aspects of the Endomorph Diet is its inclusivity. This is not a restrictive regimen that eliminates entire food groups or mandates unrealistic expectations. Instead, it encourages you to explore a diverse array of ingredients, savor the richness of whole foods, and revel in the joy of cooking. With recipes spanning cultures and cuisines, you'll discover that eating for your endomorph body type is a global celebration of nourishment.

In the pages that follow, you'll find a treasure trove of recipes tailored to your specific needs as an endomorph. Whether you're seeking breakfast inspiration to kickstart your day, vibrant salads that burst with flavor, hearty mains that satisfy both hunger and cravings, or delectable treats that offer a touch of indulgence, there's something here for every occasion. Each recipe is more than a set of instructions; it's an invitation to embark on a culinary exploration, to experiment with ingredients, and to make every meal a reflection of self-care.

To make your journey even more rewarding, this cookbook is infused with nutritional insights, cooking tips, and practical advice. You'll learn about the role of macronutrients and how they impact your endomorph body type, gaining a deeper understanding of how to make informed choices that align with your health objectives. Moreover, the emphasis on portion control empowers you to enjoy your favorite dishes while keeping your goals firmly in sight.

As you flip through these pages, remember that the Endomorph Diet is not a quick fix but a lifelong commitment to vitality. It's about progress, not perfection. Every step you take towards adopting healthier habits is a victory, and every meal you prepare from this cookbook is a testament to your dedication to yourself.

I extend my deepest gratitude to you for choosing this endomorph diet cookbook to be your companion on this transformative journey. May it inspire you to embrace the joys of cooking, savor the flavors of nourishment, and cultivate a radiant well-being that radiates from the inside out. Here's to the endless possibilities that lie ahead as you embark on a path of self-discovery, empowerment, and delicious fulfillment.

Your journey begins now. Turn the page and step into a world of discovery, transformation, and well-being. Welcome to the Endomorph Diet family – a community that celebrates diversity, honors individuality, and believes that the pursuit of health is a beautiful and empowering endeavor.

Bon appétit and best wishes on your Endomorph Diet adventure!

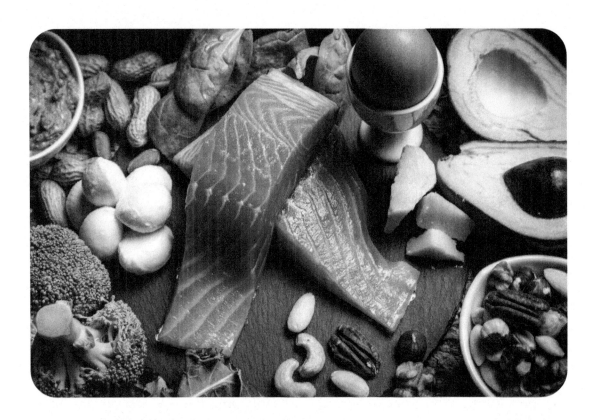

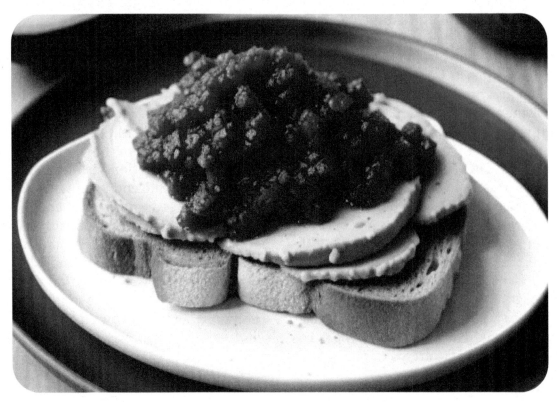

Chapter 1: Understanding Your Endomorph Body Type

Understanding Body Types

The concept of somatotypes, developed by psychologist William H. Sheldon in the 1940s, offers a lens through which we can better comprehend the remarkable diversity of human physiques. These classifications, known as body types, help categorize individuals based on their distinct physical and metabolic characteristics. While these categories provide a foundational framework, it's essential to recognize that each person's body is a unique amalgamation of traits that may span multiple somatotypes.

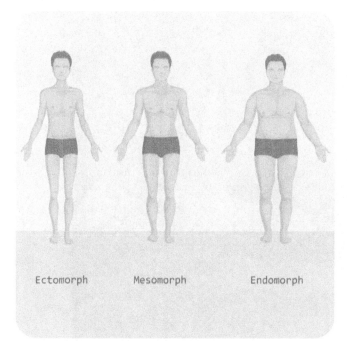

Ectomorph   Mesomorph   Endomorph

Ectomorphs: The Lean and Lithe

Ectomorphs represent those individuals who possess a lean and delicate physique. These individuals often have a slender build with a tendency towards lower body fat levels. Ectomorphs are characterized by a faster metabolism, which means they can consume a relatively higher amount of calories without gaining significant weight. This metabolic advantage, however, can also pose challenges, as ectomorphs may struggle to gain muscle mass and develop a more muscular appearance. Their narrower bone structure can contribute to a more linear body shape.

Mesomorphs: The Athletic Powerhouses

Mesomorphs exhibit a more muscular and athletic build. These individuals tend to have a naturally higher percentage of lean muscle mass, making them well-suited for activities that require strength and power. Their bodies respond more efficiently to resistance training, allowing them to gain muscle relatively easily. This muscle development is often accompanied by a more defined physique, characterized by well-sculpted muscles and a V-shaped upper body. Mesomorphs also tend to have a moderate metabolism, striking a balance between ectomorphs and endomorphs.

Endomorphs: The Soft Curves and Challenges

Endomorphs possess a rounder and softer body shape, with a predisposition to store body fat more easily. These individuals typically have a slower metabolism compared to ectomorphs and mesomorphs, which can lead to challenges in weight management. Endomorphs often find it more difficult to lose weight and may need to be more vigilant with their dietary choices. Their bodies have a greater tendency to hold onto fat reserves, which might have evolutionary advantages during periods of scarcity. The endomorph's frame tends to be fuller, and their body composition may include a mix of muscle and fat.

What Exactly is an Endomorph?

In the realm of body types and fitness, the term "endomorph" holds a significant place. Endomorphs are one of the three primary somatotypes, a classification system developed in the early 20th century to describe variations in human physique. The concept of endomorphs, alongside ectomorphs and mesomorphs, has been widely discussed in the fitness and nutrition communities to help individuals better understand their bodies and tailor their lifestyles for optimal well-being.

Defining Endomorphs:

Endomorphs are characterized by a certain set of physical and metabolic traits that distinguish them from the other somatotypes. These traits include a tendency to store more body fat, a rounder and softer appearance, a slower metabolism, and a potentially greater difficulty in losing weight compared to the other body types.

Physical Characteristics:

Endomorphs typically have a naturally curvier or stockier build. They tend to have a softer, rounder body shape, with a higher percentage of body fat. This doesn't mean that all endomorphs are overweight; rather, their bodies are predisposed to holding on to fat more easily.

Metabolic Factors:

One of the key factors associated with endomorphs is their metabolic rate. Endomorphs usually have a slower metabolism compared to mesomorphs and ectomorphs. This means

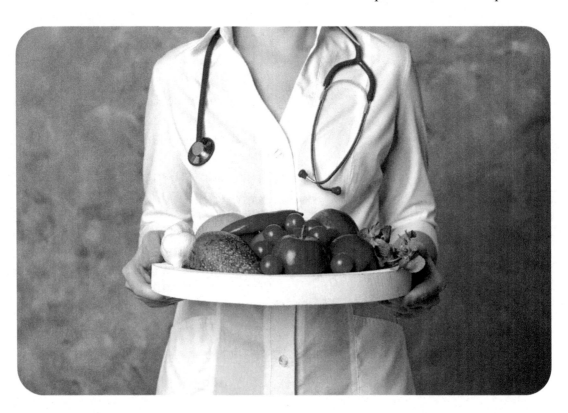

their bodies might burn calories at a slightly slower rate, which can contribute to challenges in weight management.

Challenges and Advantages:

While endomorphs might face challenges in maintaining or achieving a certain level of leanness, it's essential to note that being an endomorph comes with its own set of advantages. For instance, their naturally higher body fat percentage can provide insulation and energy reserves, which might have been advantageous for our ancestors during times of scarcity. Additionally, endomorphs often have a rounder and more approachable appearance, which can be seen as friendly and comforting.

Nutritional Considerations:

Due to their metabolic tendencies, endomorphs often need to pay closer attention to their dietary choices. A diet that is balanced and focuses on whole, nutrient-dense foods can be particularly beneficial. Carbohydrates, which are a primary source of energy, should be consumed mindfully to avoid excessive fat storage. Proteins play a crucial role in supporting muscle mass and metabolism. Healthy fats are essential for various bodily functions.

Exercise and Lifestyle:

Physical activity is a vital component of an endomorph's journey toward well-being. Incorporating a mix of cardiovascular exercises and strength training can help boost metabolism and improve body composition. Finding an exercise routine that is enjoyable and sustainable is key for long-term success.

Individual Variation:

It's important to recognize that while the somatotype classification system offers insights into general physical tendencies, individuals are unique and can exhibit a combination of traits from different body types. Very few people fit perfectly into one somatotype category, and this diversity should be celebrated.

Embracing Wellness:

The concept of endomorphs underscores the beauty of human diversity. Each body type has its strengths and areas of growth. Rather than striving for an unrealistic ideal, the focus should be on promoting health, vitality, and overall well-being. Understanding your body type, such as being an endomorph, can provide valuable information to help you make informed choices that align with your goals.

Physical Characteristics of Endomorphs

The endomorph body type is characterized by a unique set of physical traits that distinguish it from other somatotypes. These characteristics encompass a range of attributes that influence appearance, metabolism, and overall body composition. While every individual is unique, understanding these physical traits can offer insights into how endomorphs may respond to different lifestyle choices, exercise routines, and nutritional approaches.

Body Shape

Endomorphs typically have a softer and rounder body shape. They tend to have a higher percentage of body fat, particularly in areas such as the abdomen, hips, and thighs. This can result in a curvier and fuller figure compared to other body types.

Fat Storage Tendency

One of the most distinctive characteristics of endomorphs is their tendency to store fat more easily. Their bodies are genetically predisposed to accumulate and retain fat. This evolutionary trait may have provided an advantage in times of food scarcity when energy reserves were vital for survival.

Slower Metabolism

Endomorphs often have a slower metabolic rate compared to other somatotypes. This means that their bodies burn calories at a slower pace, making it easier to gain weight if caloric intake exceeds expenditure. This metabolic tendency can present challenges in weight management and requires a more thoughtful approach to diet and exercise.

Muscle Mass

Endomorphs tend to have a natural predisposition for retaining muscle mass. While they may not gain muscle as quickly as mesomorphs, their bodies have the capacity to maintain muscle even during periods of weight loss. This can be advantageous for overall body strength and function.

Bone Structure

Endomorphs often have a broader and more robust bone structure. This can contribute to a more solid appearance and can be accompanied by a naturally heavier overall weight compared to other body types.

Challenges in Weight Loss

Due to their higher body fat percentage and slower metabolism, endomorphs may face challenges in losing weight. It might take longer and require more effort for them to achieve significant weight loss compared to other somatotypes. However, with consistent efforts and a balanced approach, sustainable progress is achievable.

Rounded Features

Endomorphs may exhibit softer and more rounded facial features. This can contribute to a youthful and approachable appearance.

Clothing Fit

Because of their curvier and fuller body shape, endomorphs may find that certain clothing styles fit them differently than individuals with other body types. Embracing styles that flatter their unique shape can enhance confidence and self-esteem.

Energy Reserves

Endomorphs naturally store more energy in the form of body fat. While excessive body fat can pose health risks, moderate fat storage can provide the body with energy reserves to draw upon during periods of increased physical activity or reduced caloric intake.

Wellness Potential

It's important to note that being an endomorph does not determine one's overall health or fitness potential. With the right strategies, endomorphs can achieve and maintain a healthy weight, enhance their fitness levels, and enjoy optimal well-being.

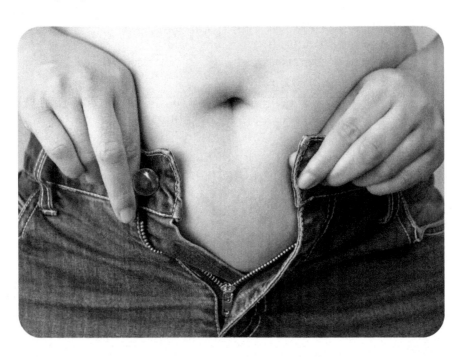

Chapter 2: The Foundations of the Endomorph Diet

What is the Endomorph Diet?

The Endomorph Diet is a personalized approach to nutrition that caters specifically to individuals with the endomorph body type. Endomorphs are characterized by their natural tendency to store body fat more easily, a rounder physique, and a potentially slower metabolism. This unique body composition calls for a tailored dietary strategy that takes into account the individual's genetic predisposition, metabolism, and overall wellness goals.

Core Principles of the Endomorph Diet:

Balanced Macronutrients

The Endomorph Diet emphasizes a balanced intake of macronutrients—carbohydrates, proteins, and fats. While the exact ratio may vary based on individual needs and activity levels, the goal is to avoid extreme restrictions or over-consumption of any particular nutrient group.

Mindful Carbohydrate Intake

Endomorphs are encouraged to be mindful of their carbohydrate intake, particularly refined and processed carbohydrates. Focusing on complex carbohydrates from whole grains, fruits, and vegetables can help manage blood sugar levels and prevent excessive fat storage.

Portion Control

Given the endomorph body type's predisposition to weight gain, portion control plays a vital role. Monitoring portion sizes helps prevent

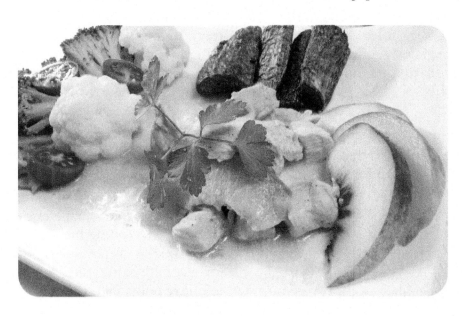

overeating and supports weight management goals.

Whole Foods

The Endomorph Diet advocates for whole, nutrient-dense foods as the foundation of a healthy diet. These foods provide essential vitamins, minerals, and fiber while promoting satiety and overall well-being.

Lean Proteins

Adequate protein intake is crucial for maintaining muscle mass and supporting metabolic function. Lean protein sources like poultry, fish, beans, and legumes are recommended.

Healthy Fats

Including healthy fats from sources such as avocados, nuts, seeds, and olive oil provides essential fatty acids and supports various bodily functions.

Sample Dietary Guidelines for Endomorphs:

Breakfast

Start the day with a balanced breakfast that includes protein, complex carbohydrates, and healthy fats. This could be a vegetable omelet with whole-grain toast or Greek yogurt with berries and nuts.

Lunch

Opt for a satisfying lunch that combines lean protein, colorful vegetables, and a moderate amount of whole grains. A grilled chicken salad with mixed greens, quinoa, and a light vinaigrette is a great choice.

Snacks

Choose nutrient-rich snacks that keep you energized between meals. Options include carrot sticks with hummus, a small handful of nuts, or a piece of fruit with a slice of cheese.

Dinner

Enjoy a well-balanced dinner featuring lean protein, plenty of vegetables, and a small portion of complex carbohydrates. Grilled salmon with steamed broccoli and brown rice is a wholesome option.

Hydratio

Stay hydrated by drinking plenty of water throughout the day. Herbal teas and infused water are also great choices.

Limit Added Sugars

Minimize your intake of sugary beverages, sweets, and processed foods that contain added sugars.

Customization and Sustainability:

One of the key strengths of the Endomorph Diet is its focus on individualization. While the core principles provide a framework, the diet can be customized to suit personal preferences, cultural backgrounds, and dietary restrictions. This flexibility makes it easier to adhere to the diet in the long term, promoting sustainable lifestyle changes.

Supplements for the Endomorph Diet

The Endomorph Diet emphasizes balanced nutrition and mindful eating as fundamental components of supporting the unique needs of individuals with endomorph body types. While obtaining essential nutrients primarily from whole foods is the cornerstone of this approach, there are instances where supplements can play a beneficial role in enhancing nutritional support. Here's a look at some supplements that endomorphs may consider incorporating into their wellness regimen.

Multivitamins

A high-quality multivitamin can provide a comprehensive blend of essential vitamins and minerals. Endomorphs, like anyone else, may occasionally fall short in meeting their daily nutrient requirements due to dietary limitations or lifestyle factors. A multivitamin can act as an insurance policy to bridge potential nutritional gaps.

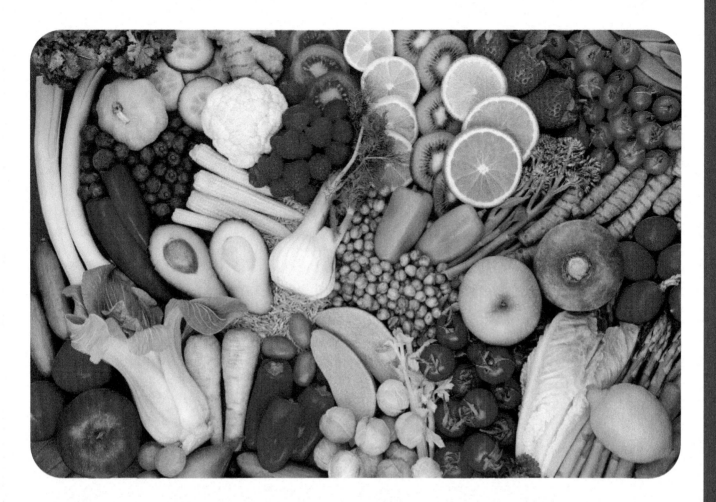

Omega-3 Fatty Acids

Omega-3 fatty acids, commonly found in fish oil supplements, offer numerous health benefits. They support cardiovascular health, help manage inflammation, and contribute to optimal brain function. Given that endomorphs may have a predisposition to weight management challenges, omega-3 supplementation can aid in promoting overall well-being.

Protein Supplements

Protein is vital for maintaining muscle mass and promoting satiety. Endomorphs who engage in regular physical activity and strength training may benefit from protein supplements like whey protein or plant-based options. These supplements can assist in meeting protein needs, especially during periods of increased exercise or when dietary protein intake is insufficient.

Vitamin D

Vitamin D is essential for bone health, immune function, and overall well-being. Endomorphs, like many individuals, may have limited sun exposure, which is a primary source of vitamin D synthesis. Supplementing with vitamin D can help ensure adequate levels and support various bodily functions.

Fiber Supplements

Fiber plays a crucial role in promoting digestive health and supporting weight management. Endomorphs seeking to manage their weight more effectively may consider fiber supplements, which can aid in satiety and regulating digestion.

Magnesium

Magnesium is involved in numerous biochemical reactions in the body, including those related to metabolism and energy production.

It can also support relaxation and quality sleep, which are essential aspects of overall well-being.

B Vitamins

B vitamins, such as B6, B12, and folate, are important for energy metabolism and cognitive function. Incorporating a B-complex supplement can be beneficial, especially if dietary intake is suboptimal.

Greens Powders

Greens powders are concentrated blends of vegetables, fruits, and other plant-based ingredients. They provide a convenient way to boost nutrient intake, particularly for individuals who may struggle to consume sufficient servings of fruits and vegetables.

Prebiotics and Probiotics

Gut health is increasingly recognized as crucial for overall well-being. Prebiotic supplements support the growth of beneficial gut bacteria, while probiotics introduce live microorganisms that can positively impact digestion and immunity.

What to Avoid on the Endomorph Diet

The Endomorph Diet is a tailored approach to nutrition that takes into consideration the unique needs of individuals with the endomorph body type. This body type is characterized by a tendency to store body fat more easily, a rounder physique, and potentially slower metabolism. To promote optimal wellness and support weight management goals, there are certain foods and dietary practices that endomorphs should consider avoiding. By making mindful choices and steering clear of these potential pitfalls, individuals can enhance their journey toward well-being.

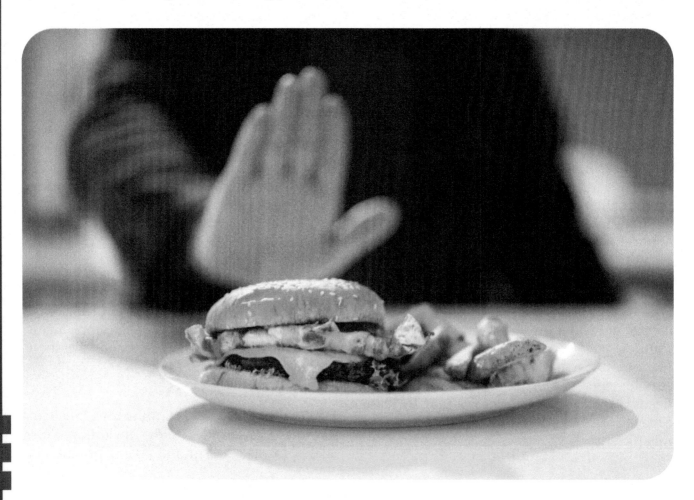

Refined Carbohydrates

Endomorphs should be cautious when it comes to refined carbohydrates such as white bread, sugary cereals, pastries, and sugary snacks. These foods can lead to rapid spikes in blood sugar levels, followed by crashes that can trigger cravings and overeating. Opting for complex carbohydrates from whole grains, fruits, and vegetables provides sustained energy and better supports blood sugar control.

Excessive Sugars

Foods high in added sugars, such as sugary beverages, candies, and desserts, should be minimized. Excess sugar consumption can contribute to weight gain, inflammation, and other health issues. Natural sources of sugar, such as fruits, can be included in moderation due to their fiber content and nutritional benefits.

Processed and Fried Foods

Processed and fried foods often contain unhealthy trans fats, excessive sodium, and artificial additives. These factors can hinder weight management efforts and compromise overall health. Opt for whole, unprocessed foods prepared using healthier cooking methods like baking, grilling, steaming, or sautéing.

High-Calorie, Low-Nutrient Foods

Foods that are high in calories but lacking in essential nutrients should be limited. These include foods like fast food, deep-fried snacks, and sugary cereals. These foods can contribute to excessive calorie intake without providing the nourishment that endomorphs need to support their health and wellness goals.

Sugary Beverages

Sugary drinks such as soda, fruit juices, and sweetened teas can lead to excess calorie consumption without providing the satiety that comes from solid foods. Opt for water, herbal teas, and naturally flavored water with a squeeze of citrus or fresh herbs to stay hydrated without unnecessary added sugars.

Excessive Alcohol

Alcohol can contribute to excess calorie intake and hinder weight loss efforts. Additionally, it can impact metabolism, disrupt sleep, and affect overall health. If you choose to consume alcohol, do so in moderation and be mindful of your choices.

Overeating and Large Portions

While not a specific food item, overeating and consuming large portions can be counterproductive for endomorphs. Portion control is crucial for managing weight and avoiding excess calorie intake. Practice mindful eating, listen to your body's hunger cues, and aim to eat until you're satisfied rather than overly full.

Low-Quality Protein Sources

Choosing protein sources that are high in unhealthy fats or processed additives can compromise the nutritional quality of your diet. Opt for lean protein sources like poultry, fish, lean cuts of meat, legumes, and plant-based protein options.

Skipping Meals

Skipping meals can lead to overeating later in the day and disrupt blood sugar levels. Consistent, balanced meals and snacks throughout the day help maintain stable energy levels and support metabolism.

Unhealthy Snacking

Opt for nutrient-dense snacks instead of reaching for empty-calorie options. Avoid chips, sugary snacks, and heavily processed snacks. Instead, choose options like whole fruit, nuts, Greek yogurt, or cut vegetables with hummus.

Chapter 3: Navigating Your Endomorph Wellness Journey

Active Your Body Metabolism

Metabolism is the complex set of chemical processes that fuel the body's energy needs. For individuals with the endomorph body type, who naturally have a slower metabolism, it's crucial to implement strategies that can help enhance metabolic rate and promote optimal energy expenditure. By adopting a combination of lifestyle habits, exercise routines, and dietary choices, endomorphs can effectively activate their metabolism and support their wellness goals.

Prioritize Physical Activity

Regular exercise is a cornerstone of boosting metabolism. Engaging in both cardiovascular activities and strength training can have a significant impact. Cardio workouts, such as brisk walking, jogging, cycling, and swimming, elevate heart rate and promote calorie burning. Meanwhile, strength training, including weight lifting and resistance exercises, builds lean muscle mass. Muscle tissue is metabolically active, meaning it burns more calories even at rest.

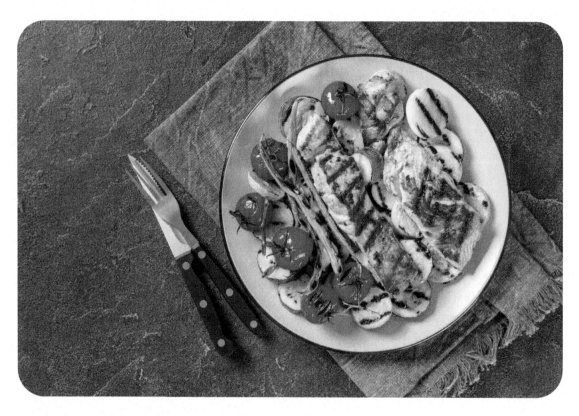

High-Intensity Interval Training (HIIT)

HIIT involves alternating between short bursts of intense exercise and periods of rest or low-intensity activity. This type of workout can elevate metabolism and promote calorie burn not only during the workout but also in the hours following. HIIT can be particularly effective for endomorphs seeking to increase their metabolic rate.

Stay Hydrated

Drinking enough water is essential for maintaining optimal metabolic function. Even mild dehydration can lead to a decrease in metabolic efficiency. Aim to drink water throughout the day and consider starting your morning with a glass of water to kickstart your metabolism.

Prioritize Protein Intake

Protein-rich foods require more energy for digestion and absorption, which can temporarily increase metabolic rate. Additionally, protein supports muscle maintenance and growth, helping to boost metabolism in the long term. Include lean protein sources like poultry, fish, legumes, and low-fat dairy in your diet.

Eat Regular Meals and Snacks

Frequent, balanced meals and snacks can prevent energy dips and help maintain stable blood sugar levels. This encourages consistent metabolic activity throughout the day. Avoid skipping meals, which can lead to metabolic slowdown.

Get Sufficient Sleep

Adequate sleep is vital for metabolic health. Poor sleep can disrupt hormonal balance and lead to a slower metabolism. Aim for 7-9 hours of quality sleep each night to support overall wellness and energy expenditure.

Manage Stress

Chronic stress can negatively impact metabolism. Stress hormones like cortisol can contribute to fat storage and hinder weight management efforts. Incorporate stress-reducing practices such as meditation, deep breathing, yoga, or spending time in nature.

Increase Non-Exercise Activity

Everyday activities like walking, taking the stairs, and household chores can contribute to calorie burn and keep metabolism active. These activities are collectively known as non-exercise activity thermogenesis (NEAT).

Don't Skip Breakfast

Starting the day with a balanced breakfast can jumpstart your metabolism. Include a mix of protein, complex carbohydrates, and healthy fats to provide sustained energy.

Stay Consistent

Consistency is key when it comes to activating and maintaining a healthy metabolism. Adopting these habits over time and making them part of your daily routine can yield sustainable results.

Endomorph Exercises

For endomorphs, exercise is not only about boosting metabolism but also about building lean muscle mass, enhancing cardiovascular health, and promoting overall strength. Tailoring your exercise routine to your body type can yield more effective and sustainable results. Here are some exercise strategies that can benefit endomorphs:

Strength Training

Incorporate regular strength training sessions to build lean muscle mass. Focus on compound exercises that engage multiple muscle groups, such as squats, deadlifts, bench presses, and rows. Lifting weights challenges your muscles and helps elevate your metabolism, even after your workout is done.

Cardiovascular Exercise

Cardio workouts are essential for cardiovascular health and calorie burn. Engage in activities

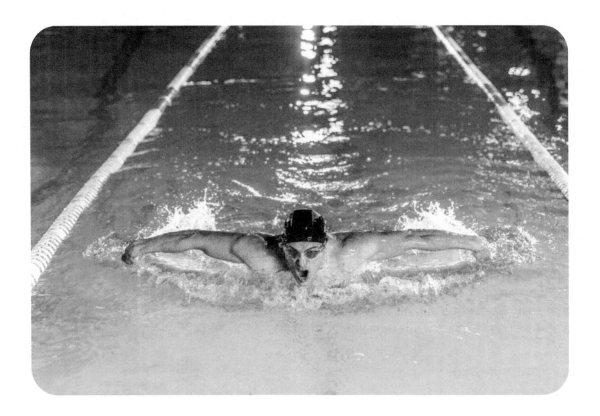

like brisk walking, jogging, cycling, swimming, or dancing. Interval training, which alternates between high-intensity bursts and recovery periods, can be particularly effective for boosting metabolism.

HIIT Workouts

High-Intensity Interval Training (HIIT) combines short bursts of intense exercise with brief recovery periods. This approach can help you burn more calories in a shorter time while improving cardiovascular fitness and boosting metabolism.

Circuit Training

Circuit training involves moving from one exercise to the next without much rest in between. It combines strength and cardio elements for an efficient and effective workout. Circuit training can help build muscle while keeping your heart rate up.

Functional Training

Functional exercises mimic movements you use in daily life. These exercises not only build strength but also improve balance, flexibility, and coordination. Examples include squats, lunges, and kettlebell swings.

Bodyweight Exercises

Bodyweight exercises use your own body as resistance. These exercises, such as push-ups, pull-ups, planks, and burpees, can be done anywhere and help build functional strength.

Core Work

A strong core is essential for stability and proper posture. Include exercises that target your core muscles, such as planks, Russian twists, and leg raises.

Flexibility and Mobility

Regular stretching and mobility exercises can help improve flexibility and prevent injuries. Yoga and Pilates are great options for promoting flexibility, balance, and overall well-being.

Active Lifestyle

Incorporate physical activity into your daily routine. Walk whenever possible, take the stairs, and find opportunities to move throughout the

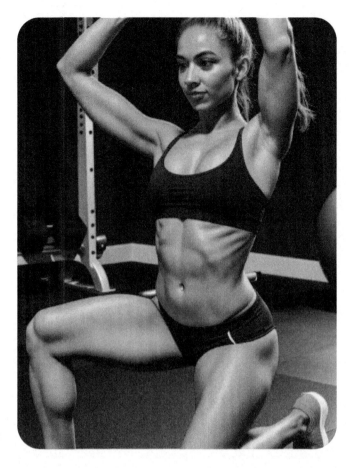

day. Non-exercise activities like gardening, playing with pets, and housecleaning also contribute to calorie burn.

Consistency and Progression

Consistency is key to achieving results. Start with manageable workout durations and gradually increase intensity and duration as your fitness improves. This progression helps prevent plateaus and keeps you motivated.

Q&As for an Effective Endomorphic Diet

Q: How can I enhance my metabolism as an endomorph?

A: To enhance metabolism, incorporate regular physical activity that includes both cardiovascular exercises and strength training. Prioritize lean protein intake, stay hydrated, get adequate sleep, and manage stress. These factors collectively contribute to boosting metabolic rate.

Q: Can I still consume carbohydrates on an endomorphic diet?

A: Yes, carbohydrates are an essential part of any diet. However, focus on complex carbohydrates from whole grains, fruits, and vegetables. These sources provide sustained energy and support stable blood sugar levels, preventing excessive fat storage.

Q: How important is portion control for endomorphs?

A: Portion control is crucial for endomorphs to prevent overeating. Be mindful of portion sizes and listen to your body's hunger and fullness cues. Eating until you're comfortably satisfied rather than overly full can support weight management.

Q: Should I avoid fats altogether on an endomorphic diet?

A: No, healthy fats are an important part of an endomorphic diet. Incorporate sources like avocados, nuts, seeds, olive oil, and fatty fish. Healthy fats provide essential nutrients, promote satiety, and support metabolic health.

Q: Can I still enjoy treats and indulge occasionally on an endomorphic diet?

A: Occasional indulgences are acceptable, but moderation is key. Treats can be incorporated into your diet without derailing your progress. It's important to maintain a balanced approach and prioritize nutrient-dense foods most of the time.

Q: Do I need to follow a strict meal plan on an endomorphic diet?

A: While meal plans can provide structure, flexibility is essential. Tailor your diet to your preferences and lifestyle. Focus on balanced meals and snacks that include lean proteins, complex carbs, healthy fats, and plenty of fruits and vegetables.

Q: How can I stay motivated and consistent with my endomorphic diet?

A: Set realistic goals, track your progress, and celebrate your successes. Surround yourself with a supportive community, engage in

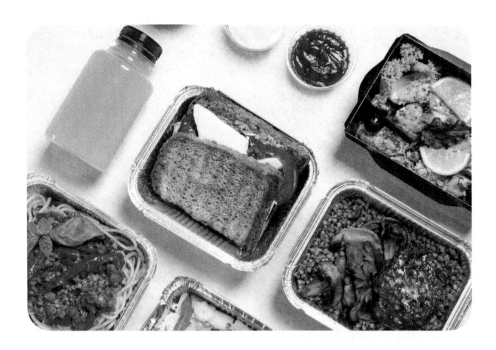

enjoyable physical activities, and experiment with new recipes to keep your diet exciting and sustainable.

Q: How can I stay on track with my endomorphic diet when dining out or traveling?

A: When dining out, choose restaurants with healthy options or review the menu ahead of time. Opt for grilled or baked dishes, choose lean proteins, and request sauces on the side. While traveling, pack nutrient-dense snacks, research dining options in advance, and focus on making balanced choices.

Q: Is it necessary to count calories on an endomorphic diet?

A: While calorie counting can be a helpful tool for some, it's not a requirement. Prioritizing whole, nutrient-dense foods and practicing portion control based on your body's hunger and fullness cues can be effective strategies for managing weight without strict calorie counting.

Q: How long does it take to see results on an endomorphic diet?

A: The timeline for seeing results varies among individuals and depends on factors such as consistency, genetics, physical activity level, and overall health. It's important to focus on progress rather than quick fixes. Small, sustainable changes over time lead to lasting results.

In conclusion, an effective endomorphic diet centers around balanced macronutrients, mindful carbohydrate choices, portion control, whole foods, and healthy fats. Prioritizing regular physical activity, staying hydrated, managing stress, and getting sufficient sleep are key to boosting metabolism. By making informed dietary choices and adopting a positive mindset, individuals with the endomorphic body type can achieve their wellness goals and maintain a strong, resilient, and healthy lifestyle.

Embrace the journey's ebb and flow, and celebrate every step you take toward becoming the healthiest version of yourself. You're not alone on this path. Join the community of individuals who, like you, are navigating their way through the intricacies of their bodies. Continue to learn, adapt, and listen to your body's whispers. The Endomorph Diet is your compass, guiding you toward a life of balance, empowerment, and wholehearted wellness. Remember, you have the power to shape your journey, and the possibilities are endless.

May your path be filled with vitality, self-discovery, and an unwavering commitment to your well-being. Embrace your unique journey and step forward with confidence, for you are the author of your health story.

Chapter 4: 28-Day Meal Plan

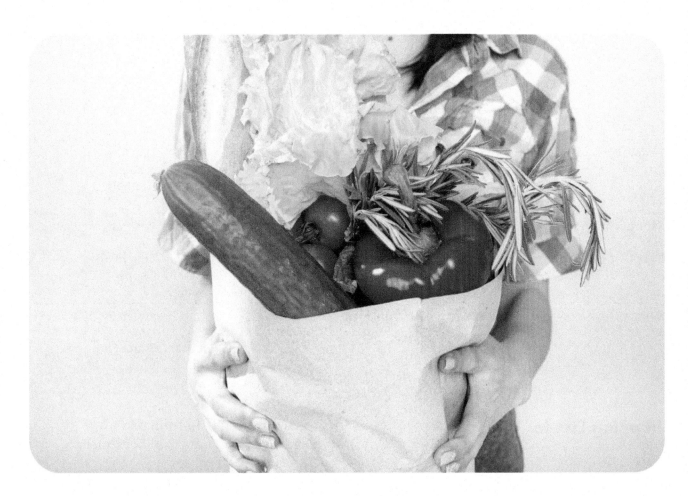

Week-1 Embracing the Journey

Welcome to Week 1 of your Endomorph Diet journey! Congratulations on taking the first step towards a healthier you. This week is all about setting the foundation for your new eating plan. Begin by focusing on portion control and balanced meals. Fill your plate with a variety of nutrient-rich foods, such as lean proteins, whole grains, and colorful vegetables.

Remember, consistency is key, so try to maintain regular meal times to stabilize your energy levels. And don't forget to stay hydrated – water plays a vital role in supporting your metabolism and curbing unnecessary snacking. As you navigate this week, keep in mind that it's about progress, not perfection. Embrace the small victories and let them fuel your determination for the weeks ahead.

DAY	CARB INTAKE	BREAKFAST	SNACK	LUNCH	SNACK	DINNER	TOTAL CARBS
Monday	High Carb	Quinoa porridge	Peanut Butter Protein Cookies	Lemon, Herb, and Cheese Pasta	Peanut Butter Protein Cookies	Haddock & Kale Crumble	174.5
Tuesday	Moderate Carb	Egg Muffin Cups	Peanut Butter Protein Cookies	Haddock & Kale Crumble	Peanut Butter Protein Cookies	Rosemary Lime Butter Pork Chops	63.2
Wednesday	Low Carb	Egg Muffin Cups	Hard-Boiled Eggs	Slow-Cooked Chicken	Raw Veggies With Ranch Dressing	Rosemary Lime Butter Pork Chops	24.2
Thursday	High Carb	Quinoa porridge	Peanut Butter Protein Cookies	Lemon, Herb, and Cheese Pasta	Peanut Butter Protein Cookies	Haddock & Kale Crumble	174.5
Friday	High Carb	Quinoa porridge	Peanut Butter Protein Cookies	Lemon, Herb, and Cheese Pasta	Peanut Butter Protein Cookies	Haddock & Kale Crumble	174.5
Saturday	Low Carb	Egg Muffin Cups	Hard-Boiled Eggs	Slow-Cooked Chicken	Raw Veggies With Ranch Dressing	Rosemary Lime Butter Pork Chops	24.2
Sunday	Low Carb	Egg Muffin Cups	Hard-Boiled Eggs	Slow-Cooked Chicken	Raw Veggies With Ranch Dressing	Rosemary Lime Butter Pork Chops	24.2

Shopping List for Week 1

Proteins:

- 1 pound boneless, skinless chicken breast
- 4 1-inch bone-in pork chops
- 4 haddock fillets, skinless & boneless
- 4 large eggs

Vegetables:

- ½ cup diced green bell pepper
- ½ cup diced red bell pepper
- 1 cup packed baby spinach, roughly chopped
- 1 clove garlic
- ½ cup diced onion
- ½ cup diced mushrooms
- ½ teaspoon organic vanilla extract
- ½ cup curly kale
- 3 carrots, sliced into sticks
- 3 celery stalks, sliced into sticks
- 1 small cucumber, sliced

Fruits:

- Fresh lemon zest

Miscellaneous:

- 2 cups of water
- ½ cup coconut milk

- 1 cup uncooked red quinoa, rinsed and drained
- 2 tablespoons almonds, chopped
- 1 (16-ounce) package penne
- ½ cup reserved pasta water
- 2 tablespoons butter
- 1 cup ricotta cheese
- 1 teaspoon ground cinnamon
- ½ teaspoon ground ginger
- ½ teaspoon ground nutmeg
- 1 tsp garlic paste or 1 clove of minced garlic
- 1 teaspoon cinnamon
- 1 teaspoon parsley
- ½ cup ranch dressing

Nuts:

- 2 tablespoons almonds, chopped

Week-2 Building Healthy Habits

You've made it to Week 2, and by now, you're starting to notice positive changes in how you feel. This week, let's focus on building healthy eating habits. Incorporate snacks into your routine to keep your metabolism active and prevent overindulging at mealtime. Opt for smart choices like Greek yogurt, mixed nuts, or sliced fruits. As you explore different foods, pay attention to how your body responds. Listen to your hunger cues and aim to eat mindfully, savoring each bite. Experiment with new recipes that align with your dietary goals – variety can make healthy eating exciting and sustainable. Remember, every step you take this week is a step towards a healthier, happier you.

DAY	CARB INTAKE	BREAKFAST	SNACK	LUNCH	SNACK	DINNER	TOTAL CARBS
Monday	High Carb	Quinoa Porridge	High-Protein Oatmeal Cookies	Taco Corn Chowder	High-Protein Oatmeal Cookies	Chipotle Chicken Bowl	168.5
Tuesday	Moderate Carb	Quinoa Porridge	High-Protein Oatmeal Cookies	Garlic Butter Baked Pork	High-Protein Oatmeal Cookies	Spicy Roasted Spaghetti Squash	78.5
Wednesday	Low Carb	Avocado Egg Tarts	Turkey Apricot Roll-Ups	Garlic Butter Baked Pork	Turkey Apricot Roll-Ups	Spicy Roasted Spaghetti Squash	20
Thursday	High Carb	Quinoa Porridge	High-Protein Oatmeal Cookies	Taco Corn Chowder	High-Protein Oatmeal Cookies	Chipotle Chicken Bowl	168.5
Friday	High Carb	Quinoa Porridge	High-Protein Oatmeal Cookies	Taco Corn Chowder	High-Protein Oatmeal Cookies	Chipotle Chicken Bowl	168.5
Saturday	Low Carb	Avocado Egg Tarts	Turkey Apricot Roll-Ups	Garlic Butter Baked Pork	Turkey Apricot Roll-Ups	Spicy Roasted Spaghetti Squash	20
Sunday	Low Carb	Avocado Egg Tarts	Turkey Apricot Roll-Ups	Garlic Butter Baked Pork	Turkey Apricot Roll-Ups	Spicy Roasted Spaghetti Squash	20

Shopping List for Week 2

Proteins:

- 3 large eggs
- 2 medium-sized pork chops
- 12 ounces of cooked and shredded chicken
- 6 (1-ounce) slices deli roasted turkey

Vegetables:

- Fresh lemon zest (for quinoa porridge)
- Toppings of your choice (for avocado egg tarts)
- 1 medium yellow onion, peeled and diced
- 1 shallot, minced
- 8 cups chopped Romaine lettuce
- Chopped fresh cilantro

Fruits:

- 3 avocados

Miscellaneous:

- 2 cups of water
- ½ cup coconut milk
- 1 cup uncooked red quinoa, rinsed and drained
- 10-12 drops of liquid stevia

- 1 tablespoon extra virgin olive oil
- 2 tablespoons unsalted butter
- 1 tablespoon apricot preserves
- 1 tablespoon dijon mustard
- 1 3/4 cups dry oats
- 1/2 cup applesauce
- Dash cinnamon

Nuts:

- 2 tablespoons almonds, chopped

Week-3 Fine-Tuning and Progressing

Welcome to Week 3, where you'll fine-tune your Endomorph Diet plan and take your commitment to the next level. This week, focus on portion sizes and optimizing your nutrient intake. Incorporate a wider range of vegetables to increase fiber content and promote better digestion. Try different cooking methods – grilling, roasting, or steaming – to enhance flavors without adding unnecessary calories. Don't forget the importance of lean proteins, as they support muscle maintenance and aid in keeping you full for longer. Reflect on your journey so far and celebrate the positive changes you've experienced. Your dedication is paying off, and you're on track to achieving your goals.

DAY	CARB INTAKE	BREAKFAST	SNACK	LUNCH	SNACK	DINNER	TOTAL CARBS
Monday	High Carb	Oatmeal With Peanut Butter & Banana	Protein Cheesecake	Salmon Fettuccini	Protein Cheesecake	Salmon Fettuccini	234
Tuesday	Moderate Carb	Low-Calorie Bacon, Egg, And Cheese	Lemon Coconut Protein Balls	Farro Salad	Lemon Coconut Protein Balls	Farro Salad	97.4
Wednesday	Low Carb	Bagel Avocado Toast	Lemon Coconut Protein Balls	Shrimp Mexicana	Lemon Coconut Protein Balls	Spicy Peanut Tempeh Salad	43.5
Thursday	High Carb	Oatmeal With Peanut Butter & Banana	Protein Cheesecake	Salmon Fettuccini	Protein Cheesecake	Salmon Fettuccini	234
Friday	High Carb	Oatmeal With Peanut Butter & Banana	Protein Cheesecake	Salmon Fettuccini	Protein Cheesecake	Salmon Fettuccini	234

DAY	CARB INTAKE	BREAKFAST	SNACK	LUNCH	SNACK	DINNER	TOTAL CARBS
Saturday	Low Carb	Bagel Avocado Toast	Lemon Coconut Protein Balls	Shrimp Mexicana	Lemon Coconut Protein Balls	Spicy Peanut Tempeh Salad	43.5
Sunday	Low Carb	Bagel Avocado Toast	Lemon Coconut Protein Balls	Shrimp Mexicana	Lemon Coconut Protein Balls	Spicy Peanut Tempeh Salad	43.5

Shopping List for Week 3

Proteins:

- 6 egg whites
- 12 ounces fresh salmon fillets
- 24 ounces fat-free cream cheese
- 1 lb. medium shrimp peeled and deveined

Vegetables:

- 3 bananas, sliced
- 1 slice cooked turkey bacon
- ½ medium avocado, peeled, mashed
- 2 cloves garlic
- 3 cups chopped kale
- 3 cups packed baby arugula
- ¼ cup thinly sliced fresh basil leaves
- 2 whole, canned artichoke hearts, rinsed, chopped

Fruits:

- 3 bananas
- 1 lime
- 3 tablespoons pomegranate seeds or dried cranberries
- 4 tablespoons lemon juice
- ½ teaspoon grated lemon zest

Miscellaneous:

- 2 cups old-fashioned oats
- 2-3 tablespoons everything bagel seasoning
- Sea salt and pepper
- 1 tablespoon clarified butter
- 2 tablespoons natural peanut butter

- 2 tablespoons white wine vinegar
- Pinch ground cayenne pepper
- 2 tablespoons lemon juice
- 2 scoops vanilla whey protein
- ¾ cup stevia
- 1 teaspoon vanilla extract
- 2 tablespoons honey
- 2 tablespoons coconut flour

Nuts:

- 2 tablespoons almonds, chopped
- ¼ cup chopped, salted, roasted pistachio nuts

Week-4 Sustaining Success

Congratulations, you've reached Week 4, the final stretch of the Endomorph Diet's eating plan! This week is all about sustaining the habits you've developed over the past few weeks. Continue to prioritize balanced meals, portion control, and mindful eating. By now, you've likely found your favorite healthy recipes and snacks that satisfy your cravings. Remember that setbacks may occur, but they're just temporary bumps on your journey. Stay committed and focused on your long-term goals. Reflect on how far you've come and the positive impact these changes have had on your overall well-being. As you wrap up this month, take pride in your accomplishments and use them as a strong foundation for maintaining a healthy lifestyle moving forward. Your dedication to yourself is truly inspiring!

DAY	CARB INTAKE	BREAKFAST	SNACK	LUNCH	SNACK	DINNER	TOTAL CARBS
Monday	High Carb	Chocolate Banana Protein Pancakes	Chocolate Banana Cups	Calamari & Shrimp Paella	Chocolate Banana Cups	Artichoke and Olive Pasta	176
Tuesday	Moderate Carb	Chocolate Banana Protein Pancakes	Almonds & Zucchini Smoothie	Super Human Mackerel & Brawny Beetroot	Almonds & Zucchini Smoothie	Calamari & Shrimp Paella	85
Wednesday	Low Carb	Walnut and Almond Porridge 9.6	Mint Chocolate Chip Smoothie	Super Human Mackerel & Brawny Beetroot	Almonds & Blueberries Smoothie	Chicken and Vegetable Skewers	36.6
Thursday	High Carb	Chocolate Banana Protein Pancakes	Chocolate Banana Cups	Calamari & Shrimp Paella	Chocolate Banana Cups	Artichoke and Olive Pasta	176
Friday	High Carb	Chocolate Banana Protein Pancakes	Chocolate Banana Cups	Calamari & Shrimp Paella	Chocolate Banana Cups	Artichoke and Olive Pasta	176
Saturday	Low Carb	Walnut and Almond Porridge	Mint Chocolate Chip Smoothie	Super Human Mackerel & Brawny Beetroot	Almonds & Blueberries Smoothie	Chicken and Vegetable Skewers	36.6
Sunday	Low Carb	Walnut and Almond Porridge	Mint Chocolate Chip Smoothie	Super Human Mackerel & Brawny Beetroot	Almonds & Blueberries Smoothie	Chicken and Vegetable Skewers	36.6

Shopping List for Week 4

Proteins:

- 4 large egg whites
- 8 oz smoked mackerel fillets, skin removed
- 6 oz frozen cooked shrimp
- 1 lb. (450g) boneless, skinless chicken breasts

Vegetables:

- 2 medium bananas
- 1 red onion
- 1 green bell pepper
- 1 yellow onion
- 1 zucchini
- 3 cloves garlic
- 2 shallots

- 10 ounces frozen artichoke hearts, defrosted
- Fresh Italian parsley
- 1 cup halved large, oil-cured green olives
- 10 ounces fresh linguine
- 1 cup fresh Kale leaves
- 1 cup of zucchini, cooked and mashed

Fruits:

- 2 medium bananas
- 1 cup fresh blueberries
- Fresh juice of 1 lemon

Miscellaneous:

- 1 cup dry quick oats
- 2 tablespoons chocolate chips
- Sugar or artificial sweetener (optional)

- ¼ cup sunflower seeds
- ¼ cup chia seeds
- ¼ cup coconut flakes
- 4 cups almond milk
- ½ teaspoon cinnamon powder
- ¼ teaspoon ginger powder
- 1 teaspoon powdered stevia
- 1 tablespoon almond butter
- 2 tbsp olive oil
- 1 tsp caraway seeds
- 1 tsp paprika
- 1 tsp chili flakes
- 1 tbsp oregano
- 1 cup cooked brown rice

- 1/2 cup frozen peas
- 2 cups skim milk
- 3 cups cold water
- Fresh juice of 1 lemon
- 1 1/2 cups almond milk
- 1 tbsp almond butter (plain, unsalted)
- 1 tsp pure almond extract
- 2 tbsp plain yogurt (optional)
- 2 tablespoons chocolate chips

Nuts:

- ½ cup pecans
- 3 cups almonds

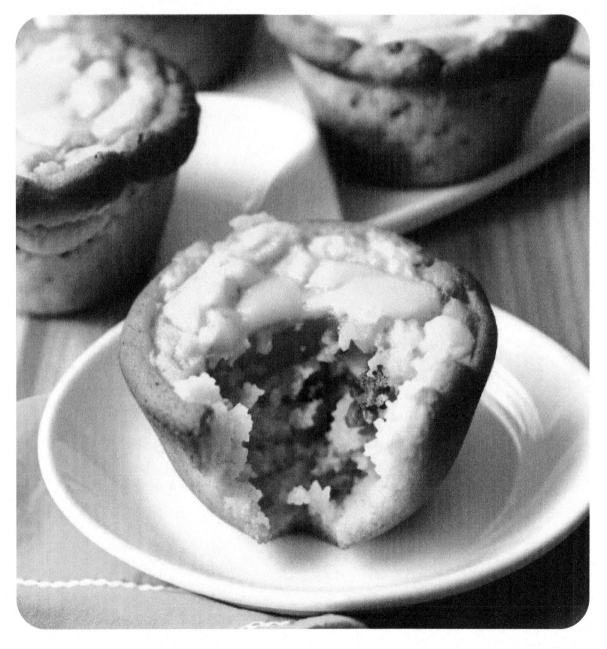

Chapter 5: Breakfast

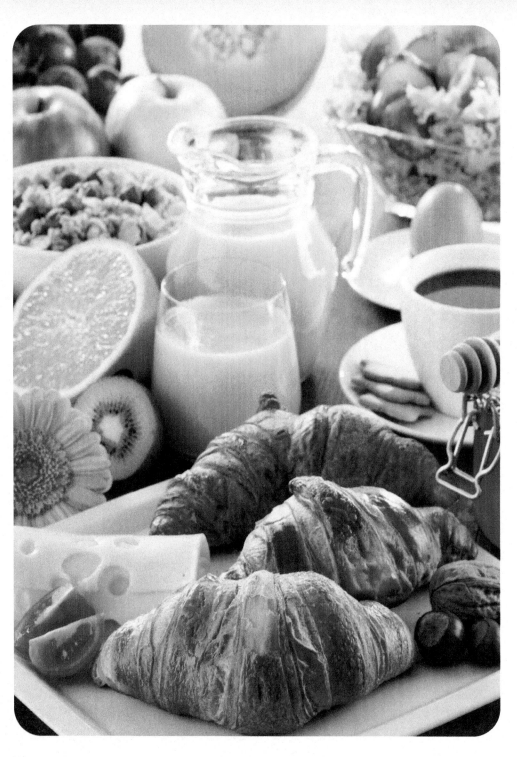

Chocolate Banana Protein Pancakes

Prep time: 5 minutes | Cook time: 2 minutes | Serves 4

- 1 cup dry quick oats
- 2 medium bananas, mashed
- 4 large egg whites
- 2 tablespoon chocolate chips
- Sugar or artificial sweetener, to taste (optional)

Steps:
1. In a medium bowl, combine oats, banana, egg whites, and chocolate chips.
2. Pour even portions of the mix onto a griddle or heated nonstick pan heated over medium heat.
3. When mix begins to bubble and set, roughly 2 minutes per side, flip over.
4. After removed from pan, pancake can be eaten as is or topped with whatever you like.

Per Serving
Calories: 192 | Fat: 3g | Protein: 7g | Sodium: 57mg | Fiber: 4g | Carbohydrates: 35g | Sugar: 14g

Walnut and Almond Porridge

Prep time: 7 minutes | Cook time: 20 minutes | Serves 5

- ½ cup pecans
- ¼ cup sunflower seeds
- ¼ cup chia seeds
- ½ cup almonds
- ¼ cup coconut flakes
- 4 cups almond milk
- ½ teaspoon cinnamon powder
- ¼ teaspoon ginger powder
- 1 teaspoon powdered stevia
- 1 tablespoon almond butter

Steps:
1. Combine pecans, almonds, and sunflower seeds in a food blender.
2. Boil the nut mixture for about 20 minutes while adding the chia seeds, coconut pieces, almond milk, spices, and stevia powder.
3. Add a spoonful of almond butter before serving.

Per Serving
Calories: 292 | Fat: 7.5g | Carbs: 9.6g | Sodium 75mg | Sugars: 1.2g | Protein: 8g

Avocado Egg Tarts

Prep time: 5 minutes | Cook time: 20 minutes | Serves 3

- 3 avocados, halved lengthwise, pitted
- 3 large eggs
- Salt and pepper to taste
- Toppings of your choice (optional)

Steps:
1. Do not peel the avocados.
2. Preheat the oven to 425 °F.
3. Put the avocado halves in a baking dish with the skin side down.
4. In each avocado cavity, crack an egg. Place the baking dish in the oven and bake until the eggs are cooked, as per your preference.
5. Sprinkle salt and pepper on top.
6. Place the toppings if using and serve.

Per Serving
Calories: 223 | Fat: 18 g | Carbohydrates: 8 g | Sugar: 0.7 g | Protein: 7 g

Bagel Avocado Toast

Prep time: 5 minutes | Cook time: 2-3 minutes | Serves 3

- ½ medium avocado, peeled, mashed
- 4 teaspoons of everything bagel seasoning
- 3 slices whole-grain bread
- Flake sea salt to garnish

Steps:
1. Toast the bread slices to the desired crispiness. Smear the mashed avocado on the bread slices.
2. Sprinkle 2 teaspoons of seasoning on each toast. Garnish with salt and serve.

Per Serving
Calories: 171 | Fat: 10.9 g | Carbohydrates: 17 g | Sugar: 2 g | Protein: 5.2 g

Two-Minute Chocolate Strawberry Protein Bowl

Prep time: 5 minutes | Cook time: none | Serves 1

- 1 cup nonfat plain Greek yogurt
- 1 cup fresh or frozen sliced strawberries
- 1–2 tablespoons dark chocolate chunks
- 2 tablespoons sugar-free chocolate syrup
- 1 scoop chocolate whey protein powder (optional)

Steps:
1. In a medium bowl, combine all ingredients and mix.
2. The whey protein is optional, but an easy way to get an extra 20–25 grams of protein into your daily intake.

Per Serving
Calories: 434 | Fat: 11g | Protein: 40g | Sodium: 215mg | Fiber: 9g | Carbohydrates: 46g | Sugar: 35g

Greek Yogurt with Mixed Berries & Almonds

Prep time: 5 minutes | Cook time: none | Serves 2

- 2 cups plain Greek yogurt
- 1 cup mixed berries (such as strawberries, blueberries, and raspberries)
- ¼ cup sliced almonds
- 2 tablespoons honey (optional)

Steps:
1. Mix the Greek yogurt, mixed berries, and sliced almonds in a bowl.
2. Drizzle with honey (optional).
3. Serve and enjoy!

Per Serving
Calories: 360 | Fat: 18g | Protein: 30g | Carbs: 26g | Fiber: 4g

Quinoa Porridge

Prep time: 7 minutes |Cook time: 15 minutes |Serves 4

- 2 cups of water
- ½ teaspoon organic vanilla extract
- pinch of ground cloves
- ½ cup coconut milk
- 1 cup uncooked red quinoa rinsed and drained
- ¼ teaspoon fresh lemon zest finely grated
- 10-12 drops of liquid stevia
- 1 teaspoon ground cinnamon
- ½ teaspoon ground ginger
- ½ teaspoon ground nutmeg
- 2 tablespoons almonds chopped

Per Serving
Calories: 248 | Fat: 11.4g | Carbohydrates: 30.5g | Protein: 7.4g

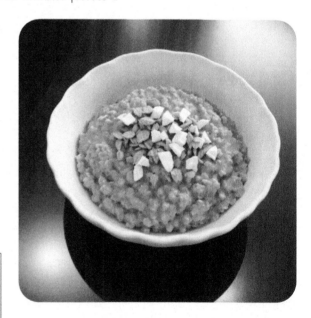

Steps:
1. In a skillet, combine the quinoa, water, and vanilla essence. Bring to a boil.
2. Lower the heat to a simmering level for roughly 15 minutes.
3. Toss the quinoa in the skillet with coconut milk, lemon zest, stevia, and seasonings.
4. Take the quinoa off the fire and immediately fluff it with a fork.
5. Evenly distribute the quinoa mixture among the serving dishes.
6. Garnish with chopped nuts when serving.

Oatmeal with Almond Milk, Chia Seeds & Banana

Prep time: 5 minutes | Cook time: 5 minutes | Serves 2

- 1 cup rolled oats
- 2 cups almond milk
- 1 ripe banana, sliced
- 1 tbsp chia seeds
- Sweetener of choice (optional)

Steps:
1. In a medium saucepan, bring the almond milk to a boil.
2. Add the rolled oats and stir to combine.
3. Reduce heat to low and let simmer for about 5 minutes or until the oats are fully cooked.
4. Remove from heat and stir in the chia seeds.
5. Serve the oatmeal in a bowl and top with sliced bananas.
6. If desired, sweeten with your preferred sweetener.

Per Serving
Calories: 280 | Fat: 8g | Protein: 8g | Carbs: 47g | Fiber: 8g

Oatmeal with Peanut Butter & Banana

Prep time: 5 minutes | Cook time: 5 minutes | Serves 3

- 2 cups old-fashioned oats
- 3 cups water
- 3 bananas, sliced
- 3 tbsp natural peanut butter

Steps:
1. In a saucepan, bring 2 cups of water to a boil.
2. Add the oats and reduce the heat to a simmer. Cook for 5 minutes or until fully cooked.
3. In a bowl, add the cooked oatmeal and top with sliced bananas and peanut butter. Enjoy!

Per Serving
Calories: 400 | Fat: 15g | Protein: 20g | Carbs: 60g

Egg Muffin Cups

Prep time: 10 minutes | Cook time: 15 minutes | Serves 4

- ½ tablespoon olive oil
- ½ cup diced green bell pepper
- ½ cup diced red bell pepper
- 1 cup packed baby spinach, roughly chopped
- 1 clove garlic, minced
- ½ cup diced onion
- ½ cup diced mushrooms
- 2 large egg whites
- 2 large eggs
- Salt to taste
- Hot sauce to serve

Steps:
1. Preheat the oven to 425 °F. Coat a 6-count muffin pan with a generous amount of oil or use cooking spray.
2. Over medium heat, heat a nonstick pan. Pour oil into the pan and wait for it to heat.
3. Add the onion and the bell peppers into the hot oil and stir. Stir often until the veggies are tender.
4. Stir in the mushrooms and spinach and cook for a couple of minutes.
5. Add the garlic and mix well. Cook for about 30 seconds, stirring often.
6. Turn off the heat and add salt to taste. Let it cool for 5-7 minutes.
7. Combine the eggs and egg whites in a bowl and whisk well.
8. Add the sautéed vegetables and stir.
9. Divide the mixture into the muffin pan. Place the muffin pan in the oven and bake until the eggs are set (for about 20 minutes).
10. Cool and drizzle hot sauce on top and serve.

Per Serving
Calories: 52 | Fat: 2.3 g | Carbohydrates: 3.2 g | Sugar: 0.8 g | Protein: 5.4 g

Low-Calorie Bacon, Egg, and Cheese

Prep time: 5 minutes | Cook time: none | Serves 1

- 1 whole-grain English muffin
- 1 large whole egg
- 1/4 teaspoon salt
- 1/8 teaspoon ground black pepper
- 1 slice cooked turkey bacon
- 1 slice fat-free cheese

Steps:
1. Slice English muffin and place in a toaster.
2. While it is toasting, cook egg in a medium skillet over medium heat to your desired consistency (over easy, over medium, etc.) Add salt and pepper.
3. Place egg, cooked bacon strip, and cheese in toasted muffin and enjoy.

Per Serving
Calories: 308 | Fat: 13g | Protein: 24g | Sodium: 1,019mg | Fiber: 1g | Carbohydrates: 24g | Sugar: 2g

Chapter 6: Snacks and Drinks

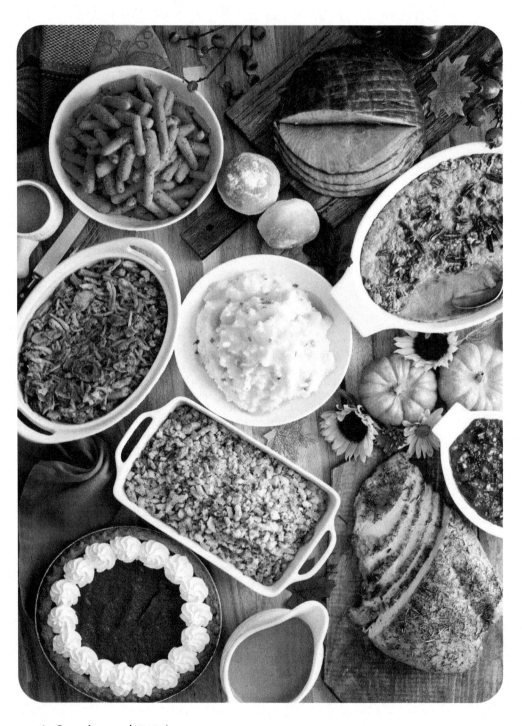

No-Bake Apple Crisp

Prep time: 5 minutes | Cook time: none | Serves 1

- 3/4 cup nonfat plain Greek yogurt
- 2 tablespoons unsweetened applesauce
- 1 medium apple, sliced or diced, peeled if desired
- Pinch stevia, or other artificial sweetener
- Pinch cinnamon
- Pinch nutmeg

Steps:
1. Mix all ingredients together in a small bowl and enjoy.

Per Serving

Calories: 220 | Fat: 7g | Protein: 7g | Sodium: 86mg | Fiber: 4g | Carbohydrates: 36g | Sugar: 28g

Cinnamon Apple Snack Bars

Prep time: 5 minutes | Cook time: 30 minutes | Serves 4

- 3/4 cup rolled oats
- 1/4 cup oat bran
- 6 large egg whites
- 1 scoop vanilla protein powder (or cinnamon swirl protein)
- 2 tablespoons unsweetened applesauce
- 1/4 teaspoon baking powder
- Pinch stevia
- Pinch cinnamon
- Drop vanilla extract
- 2 medium apples, peeled and diced

Steps:
1. Preheat oven to 350°F.
2. In a blender, combine all ingredients except apples. Blend until mixture gets thick. Pour mixture into a large bowl.
3. Add apples to mixture and stir to combine.
4. Pour mixture into 13″ × 9″ baking dish and bake 30 minutes. Cut into 4 equal bars.

Per Serving

Calories: 165 | Fat: 2g | Protein: 15g | Sodium: 124mg | Fiber: 4g | Carbohydrates: 26g | Sugar: 10g

Apple Slices with Almond Butter

Prep time: 5 minutes | Cook time: 0 minutes | Serves 2

- 2 apples, sliced
- 2 tbsp almond butter

Steps:
1. Slice the apples.
2. Spread almond butter on each apple slice.
3. Enjoy as a snack.

Per Serving

Calories: 250 | Fat: 20g | Protein: 5g | Carbs: 25g

Raw Veggies with Hummus

Prep time: 10 minutes | Cook time: 0 minutes | Serves 2

- 2 cups mixed raw veggies (e.g. carrot sticks, cherry tomatoes, cucumber slices)
- ½ cup hummus

Steps:
1. Wash and prepare the raw veggies.
2. Serve the veggies with hummus for dipping.

Per Serving

Calories: 200 | Fat: 14g | Protein: 6g | Carbs: 14g | Fiber: 6g

Mint Chocolate Chip Smoothie

Prep time: 5 minutes | Cook time: none | Serves 3

- 3 scoops chocolate protein powder
- 3 teaspoons mint extract
- 2 cups skim milk
- 3 cups cold water
- 3 teaspoons cocoa powder
- Pinch stevia
- 8 ice cubes

Steps:
1. Combine all ingredients in a blender and process until smooth.
2. Serve immediately.

Per Serving

Calories: 160 | Fat: 2g | Protein: 29g | Sodium: 101mg | Fiber: 1g | Carbohydrates: 8g | Sugar: 7g

Raw Veggies with Ranch Dressing

Prep time: 10 minutes | Cook time: none | Serves 3

- 3 carrots, sliced into sticks
- 3 celery stalks sliced into sticks
- 1 small cucumber, sliced
- 1 small bell pepper, sliced
- ½ cup ranch dressing

Steps:
1. Wash and slice the vegetables into sticks or slices.
2. Arrange the carrots, celery, cucumber, and bell pepper on a large plate or in a serving dish.
3. Serve the raw veggies with 1/4 cup of ranch dressing for each serving.
4. Serve and enjoy!

Per Serving

Calories: 140 | Fat: 13 g | Cholesterol: 5 mg | Sodium: 550 mg | Carbohydrates: 7 g | Fiber: 2 g | Sugar: 4 g | Protein: 2 g

Hard-Boiled Eggs

Prep time: 5 minutes | Cook time: 10 minutes | Serves 4

4 large eggs

Per Serving

Calories: 140 | Total Fat: 10g | Carbohydrates: 1g | Dietary Fiber: 0g | Sugars: 1g | Protein: 12g

Steps:
1. Place the eggs in a saucepan and cover with cold water.
2. Place the saucepan over high heat and bring the water to a boil.
3. Once the water has started to boil, remove it from the heat, cover and let it sit for 10 minutes.
4. Transfer the eggs to a bowl of ice water to cool.
5. Peel the eggs and serve.

Apple Slices with Peanut Butter

Prep time: 5 minutes | Cook time: none | Serves 2

- 2 medium apples, sliced
- 2 tbsp of peanut butter

Steps:
1. Slice the apples into thin rounds and place them on a plate.
2. Spread one tablespoon of peanut butter on each slice of apple.
3. Serve immediately and enjoy the sweet and nutty flavor combination.

Per Serving

Calories: 200 | Fat: 13g | Cholesterol: 0mg | Sodium: 95mg | Carbohydrates: 18g | Fiber: 3g | Sugar: 14g | Protein: 7g

Almonds & Blueberries Smoothie

Prep time: 5 minutes | Cook time: 0 minutes | Serves 3

- 1/4 cup of ground almonds, unsalted
- 1 cup of fresh blueberries
- Fresh juice of 1 lemon
- 1 cup of fresh Kale leaves
- 1/2 cup of coconut water
- 1 cup of water
- 2 tbsp. of plain yogurt (optional)

Steps:
1. Put all the ingredients in your high-speed blender, and blend until your smoothie is smooth.
2. Pour the mixture into a chilled glass.
3. Serve and enjoy!

Per Serving
Calories: 110 | Carbohydrates: 8g | Proteins: 2g | Fat: 7g | Fiber: 2g

Tropical Blend Smoothie

Prep time: 5 minutes | Cook time: none | Serves 1

- 1 scoop vanilla protein powder
- 1 medium banana
- 1/2 cup fresh pineapple
- 1/2 cup orange juice
- 1/2 cup pineapple juice
- Pinch stevia
- 5 ice cubes

Steps:
1. Combine all ingredients in a blender and process until smooth.
2. Serve immediately.

Per Serving
Calories: 378 | Fat: 1g | Protein: 28g | Sodium: 47mg | Fiber: 5g | Carbohydrates: 69g | Sugar: 46g

Apple Slices with Cinnamon

Prep time: 5 minutes | Cook time: 0 minutes | Serves 2

- 4 medium apples, sliced
- 2 tsp cinnamon
- 2 tsp honey

Steps:
1. Slice the apples into thin pieces and place them on a plate.
2. In a small bowl, mix together the cinnamon and honey.
3. Spoon the cinnamon-honey mixture over the apple slices, making sure each slice is coated.
4. Serve immediately and enjoy!

Per Serving
Calories: 140 | Total Fat: 0g | Cholesterol: 0mg | Sodium: 0mg | Total Carbohydrates: 36g | Dietary Fiber: 4g | Sugar: 30g | Protein: 1g

Almonds & Zucchini Smoothie

Prep time: 5 minutes | Cook time: 0 minutes | Serves 2

- 1 cup of zucchini, cooked and mashed - unsalted
- 1 1/2 cups of almond milk
- 1 tbsp. of almond butter (plain, unsalted)
- 1 tsp. of pure almond extract
- 2 tbsp. of ground almonds or Macadamia almonds
- 1/2 cup of water
- 1 cup of Ice cubes crushed (optional for serving)

Steps:
1. Put all the ingredients from the list above in your fast-speed blender; blend for 45 - 60 seconds or to taste.
2. Serve with crushed ice.

Per Serving
Calories: 322 | Carbohydrates: 6g | Proteins: 6g | Fat: 30g | Fiber: 3.5g

Chapter 7: Beef, Pork, and Poultry

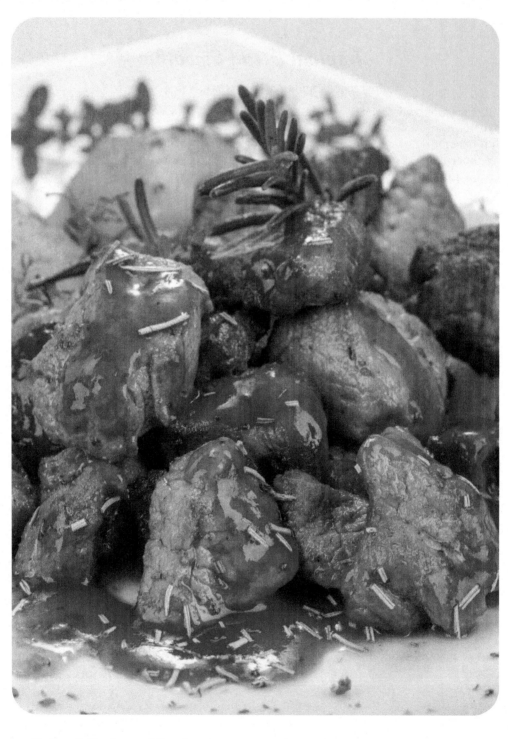

Slow-Cooked Chicken

Prep time: 5 minutes | Cook time: 4 hours | Serves 4

- 1 pound boneless, skinless chicken breast
- 1 (16-ounce) box low-sodium chicken broth
- 1 medium white onion, peeled and sliced
- 1/4 teaspoon garlic salt
- 1/8 teaspoon ground black pepper

Steps:

1. Trim and clean chicken and place in the bottom of slow cooker.
2. Pour in enough chicken broth to cover the top of the breast.
3. Add onion and seasonings to the slow cooker.
4. Cover slow cooker and cook on low setting 4 hours until chicken is done.
5. Remove and shred with a fork. It can be eaten immediately or saved for later use.

Per Serving

Calories: 199 | Fat: 5g | Protein: 27g | Sodium: 914mg | Fiber: 0g | Carbohydrates: 10g | Sugar: 1g

Chicken & Vegetable Stir-Fry

Prep time: 15 minutes | Cook time: 15 minutes | Serves 2

- 2 boneless, skinless chicken breasts sliced into thin strips
- 2 tablespoons vegetable oil
- 1 red bell pepper, sliced
- 1 yellow onion, sliced
- 1 zucchini, sliced
- 1 cup sliced mushrooms
- 1 tablespoon minced garlic
- ¼ cup low-sodium chicken broth
- 2 tablespoons low-sodium soy sauce
- 1 tablespoon cornstarch
- 2 tablespoons water
- 1 teaspoon sesame oil
- Steamed rice for serving

Steps:

1. Heat 1 tablespoon of vegetable oil in a large skillet over medium-high heat.
2. Add the chicken to the skillet and cook until browned, about 3-4 minutes. Remove the chicken from the skillet and set aside.
3. Add the remaining vegetable oil, red bell pepper, yellow onion, zucchini, and mushrooms in the same skillet. Cook until the vegetables are tender, about 5 minutes.
4. Add the garlic to the skillet and cook for 30 seconds.
5. Whisk together the chicken broth, soy sauce, cornstarch, and water in a small bowl.
6. Pour the mixture into the skillet with the vegetables and chicken and stir to combine.
7. Cook until the sauce has thickened, about 2 minutes.
8. Stir in the sesame oil.
9. Serve the chicken and vegetable stir-fry over steamed rice.

Per Serving

Calories: 427 | Fat: 21g | Cholesterol: 97mg | Sodium: 671mg | Carbohydrates: 27g | Fiber: 3g | Sugar: 6g | Protein: 38g

Chicken Parmesan

Prep time: 15 minutes | Cook time: 30 minutes | Serves 3

- 1 ½ pounds chicken breasts
- ¾ teaspoon dried minced onion
- ¾ teaspoon dried minced garlic
- ¾ teaspoon dried oregano
- ¾ teaspoon dried parsley
- ¾ teaspoon dried basil
- ⅛ teaspoon salt
- 3 ounces shredded mozzarella cheese
- ½ cup grated parmesan cheese
- 2 small eggs, beaten
- ½ cup marinara sauce from a jar
- ¼ teaspoon freshly ground black pepper

Steps:

1. First, preheat the oven to 400 °F. Place a sheet of foil on a baking sheet. Spray the foil lightly with some cooking oil spray.
2. Add the parmesan cheese, dried spices, salt, and pepper into a shallow bowl and mix well.
3. Dunk the chicken breast pieces in an egg, one at a time. Shaking off excess egg, dredge the chicken in the cheese mixture and keep it on the baking sheet.
4. When you are done with the breading, pop the baking sheet into the oven and set the timer for 20 to 25 minutes or bake until the inside temperature of the chicken is between 145 °F to 150 °F.
5. Spread the marinara sauce over the chicken. Sprinkle mozzarella on top and bake until the inside temperature of the meat shows 160 °F on the meat thermometer.
6. If you want the cheese browned, set the oven to broil mode and preheat for a few minutes.

Per Serving

Calories: 398.2 | Fat: 16.8 g | Carbohydrates: 6.5 g | Sugar: 1.9 g | Protein: 53.1 g

Pressure Cooker Beef Bourguignon

Prep time: 5 minutes | Cook time: 30 minutes | Serves 6

- 2 tablespoons unsalted butter
- 3 large onions, peeled and sliced
- 2 pounds lean beef stew meat, cubed
- 2 cups water
- 1 1/2 cups red wine
- 2 teaspoons sodium-free beef bouillon granules
- 1/2 teaspoon dried marjoram
- 1/2 teaspoon dried thyme
- 1/2 teaspoon freshly ground black pepper
- 1 pound white mushrooms, thickly sliced

Steps:

1. Melt butter in pressure cooker over medium-high heat. Add onions and cook, stirring, 5 minutes.
2. Move onions to side of pan, add cubed beef, and brown on all sides, about 5 minutes.
3. Add remaining ingredients and stir to combine. Secure the lid on the pressure cooker and set to high. Raise the heat to high and bring contents to a boil. Once you hear sizzling, reduce heat to medium and cook 20 minutes.
4. Remove from heat. Allow pressure cooker to depressurize naturally, or place under cold running water for about 5 minutes. Serve immediately.

Per Serving

Calories: 401 | Fat: 19g | Protein: 34g | Sodium: 115mg | Fiber: 2g | Carbohydrates: 12g | Sugar: 5g

Chicken and Vegetable Skewers

Prep time: 10 minutes | Cook time: 20 minutes | Serves 2-4

- 1 lb. (450g) boneless, skinless chicken breasts cut into cubes
- 1 red bell pepper, seeded and cut into chunks
- 1 green bell pepper, seeded and cut into chunks
- 1 yellow onion, peeled and cut into chunks
- 1 zucchini, cut into chunks
- 1/4 c. (60ml) olive oil
- 2 tbsp. (30ml) lemon juice
- 2 cloves garlic, minced
- 1 tsp. (5ml) dried oregano
- 1/2 tsp. (2.5ml) salt
- 1/4 tsp. (1.25ml) black pepper
- 4-6 skewers (metal or wooden)

Steps:

1. Make the marinade by whisking together the olive oil, lemon juice, garlic, oregano, salt, and black pepper in a small bowl.
2. Coat the chicken cubes in the marinade by stirring them together. Cover and refrigerate for at least 30 minutes or up to 2 hours.
3. To prevent burning on the grill, soak wooden skewers in water for at least 30 minutes if using.
4. Heat the grill to medium-high.
5. Alternate between chicken and vegetables as you thread them onto the skewers.
6. Grill the skewers for 10-15 minutes, flipping them occasionally, until the chicken is cooked through and the vegetables are tender.
7. For added flavor, garnish the chicken and vegetable skewers with fresh herbs or lemon wedges before serving.

Per Serving

Calories: 270 | Fat: 14g | Carbohydrates: 8g | Fiber: 2g | Protein: 27g

Garlic Butter Baked Pork

Prep time: 10 minutes | Cook time: 15 minutes | Serves 4

- 2 medium-sized pork chops (I like to recommend pork chops from ButcherBox because it's heritage breed pork)
- salt and pepper
- 4 tbsps. melted butter—you can also use ghee.
- 1 tbsp. fresh thyme, chopped
- 2 cloves garlic, minced
- 1 tbsp. extra virgin olive oil

Steps:

1. Preheat the oven to 375°F. Season the pork chops with salt and pepper and set aside.
2. In a small bowl, mix together the butter, thyme, and garlic. Set aside.
3. In a cast iron skillet, heat the olive oil over medium heat. When the skillet is really hot, add the pork chops. Sear until golden, about 2 minutes per side.
4. Pour the garlic butter mixture over the pork chops. Place the skillet in the oven, and cook until the pork chops reach an internal temperature of 145°F, about 10-14 minutes. The time depends on the thickness of your pork chops.
5. Remove from the oven. Using a spoon, pour some of the butter sauce left in the skillet onto the pork chops before serving.

Per Serving

Calories: 371 | Fat: 35g | Carbohydrates: 1g | Protein: 14g

Spiced Pork Chops

Prep time: 10 minutes | Cook time: 15 minutes | Serves 4

- 2 tbsps. olive oil
- 1 tbsp. Worcestershire sauce
- 1 tsp. lemon juice
- 1 tsp. paprika
- ½ tsp. onion powder
- ½ tsp. ground cumin
- ½ tsp. garlic paste
- salt and pepper
- 4 boneless pork chops

Steps:

1. In a large plastic bag add everything except for the pork. Squish it around to mix everything together.
2. Add the boneless pork chops and massage the marinade sauce around the meat.
3. Season the chops with salt and pepper on both sides and discard the sauce. Cook the chops on a preheated grill pan until cooked through, about 4-5 minutes on each side.
4. Serve with salad, horseradish coleslaw, or both!

Per Serving
Calories: 277 | Fat: 16g | Carbohydrates: 1g | Protein: 29g

Grilled Pork Tenderloin

Prep time: 10 minutes | Cook time: 15 minutes | Serves 6

- 2 whole pork tenderloin 1lb each

For The Marinade:

- ¼ cup olive oil
- ⅓ cup coconut aminos
- ¼ cup red wine vinegar
- 1 tbsp. Worcestershire sauce
- ½ juice of a lemon
- 1 tsp. dry mustard
- 1 tbsp. fresh cracked black pepper
- ½ tsp. salt
- 6 cloves garlic minced
- 1 tbsp. rosemary

Steps:

For The Marinade:

1. Combine all directions and whisk together until combined well.
2. Place tenderloins into a container or Ziplock bag and pour marinade into the bag.
3. Move around until marinade has coated tenderloins and refrigerate for up to 8 hours, but at least 2 hours before grilling.

Grilling The Pork Tenderloins:

1. Remove the tenderloins from the refrigerator one hour before grilling.
2. Heat your grill to a medium-high heat.
3. Once to temperature, add tenderloins to grill.
4. Grill tenderloins, turning every 1-2 minutes until the pork has preferred char and has reached an internal temperature of 140°F. Remove from direct heat and allow it to finish with indirect heat if needed.
5. Remove from the grill, tent with aluminum foil, and rest for 10 minutes.
6. Serve warm and enjoy!

Per Serving
Calories: 207 | Fat: 2g | Carbohydrates: 7g | Protein: 2g

Chicken & Vegetable Skewers with Quinoa

Prep time: 15 minutes | Cook time: 20-25 minutes | Serves 2

- 1 pound boneless skinless chicken breast, cut into 1-inch pieces
- 2 bell peppers, cut into 1-inch pieces
- 1 large zucchini, cut into 1-inch pieces
- 1 large yellow onion, cut into 1-inch pieces
- 1 cup cooked quinoa
- 2 tablespoons olive oil
- 1 teaspoon dried basil
- 1 teaspoon dried oregano
- Salt and pepper, to taste
- Skewers (if using wooden skewers, soak them in water for 30 minutes before using them to prevent burning)

Steps:

1. Preheat your grill to 400°F.
2. Mix the chicken, bell peppers, zucchini, onion, olive oil, basil, oregano, salt, and pepper in a large bowl.
3. Thread the chicken and vegetables onto the skewers, alternating between the chicken and the vegetables.
4. Place the skewers on the grill and cook on each side for 10-12 minutes until the chicken is cooked and the vegetables are lightly charred.
5. Serve the skewers over a bed of cooked quinoa.

Per Serving
Calories 542 | Fat: 21g | Carbohydrates: 43g | Protein: 49g | Fiber: 8g | Sodium: 209mg

Rosemary Lime Butter Pork Chops

Prep time: 10 minutes | Cook time: 15 minutes | Serves 4

- 4 1-in. cut bone-in pork chops
- salt and pepper for seasoning
- ¼ cup butter (can be melted or softened)
- 1 tbsp. chopped fresh rosemary
- 1 tbsp. lime juice
- 1 tsp. garlic paste or 1 clove of minced garlic
- ½ tsp. fresh thyme
- a pinch of red pepper flakes

Per Serving
Calories: 319 | Fat: 23g | Carbohydrates: 3g | Protein: 1g

Steps:
1. Preheat the grill. If you have a gas grill, turn it to high heat. If you have a charcoal grill, set the grill for partial direct high heat. Once the grill is hot, clean the grates by wiping them with cooking oil. Heat grill thermometer to a high heat setting
2. Generously season all sides of the pork chops with salt and pepper at least 30 minutes prior to cooking.
3. Prepare the rosemary lime butter. Add all remaining directions to a small bowl. Mix to combine.
4. Place the pork chops on the hot side of the grill about 3 inches apart and grill over direct heat for about 2 minutes each side.
5. When chops are seared on all sides, move them to indirect heat (the colder side of the grill), top with half of the rosemary lime butter and let cook for 5-6 minutes or until the internal temperature of the chops reaches 145°F. Add a dollop of combined butter mixture on top of each pork chop
6. Remove from the grill. Flip pork chops over, top with remaining butter and let rest for 10 minutes before serving.
7. Serve warm and enjoy!

Chicken Pesto Rolls

Prep time: 10 minutes | Cook time: 30 minutes | Serves 2

- 2 boneless, skinless chicken breast halves
- ½ pound medium fresh mushrooms
- ¼ cup pesto, divided
- 2 slices low-fat provolone cheese, cut into 2 halves

Per Serving
Calories: 373.4 | Fat: 17.3 g | Carbohydrates: 7.1 g | Sugar: 0.8 g | Protein: 42.4 g

Steps:
1. Preheat the oven to 350 °F. Grease a baking dish with cooking spray.
2. Chop some mushrooms and slice the other half.
3. Place the chicken breast on a sheet of plastic wrap. Pound using a meat mallet until it is uniformly about ¼ inch thick.
4. Spoon about 2 tablespoons of pesto over the chicken and spread it evenly. Scatter chopped mushrooms over the chicken. Place half cheese on each chicken.
5. Starting from the shorter end, roll the chicken and fasten it with toothpicks.
6. Scatter the sliced mushrooms on the bottom of the prepared baking dish.
7. Place the chicken rolls over the mushrooms with the seam side down. Now cover the dish with foil.
8. Place the baking dish in the oven and set the timer for about 25 minutes or until the chicken is cooked.
9. Set the oven to broil mode. Remove the foil and spread the remaining pesto over the chicken rolls. Place the remaining cheese slices on top and place them back in the oven. Broil until the cheese melts.
10. Serve.

Chipotle Chicken Bowl

Prep time: 25 minutes | Cook time: 15 minutes | Serves 4

- 12 ounces of cooked and shredded chicken
- 2 cups of whole-grain brown rice, cooked according to instructions on the package
- 8 cups of chopped Romaine lettuce
- 2 cups of tomato salsa
- Chopped fresh cilantro
- Fresh lime juice

Steps:
1. Layer ½ cup of salsa, 2 cups of lettuce, 3 ounces of chicken, and ½ cup of rice in a bowl.
2. Sprinkle lime juice and top with cilantro.

Per Serving
Calories: 246 | Carbs: 29 g | Protein: 28 g | Fat: 5 g

Chapter 8: Fish and Seafood

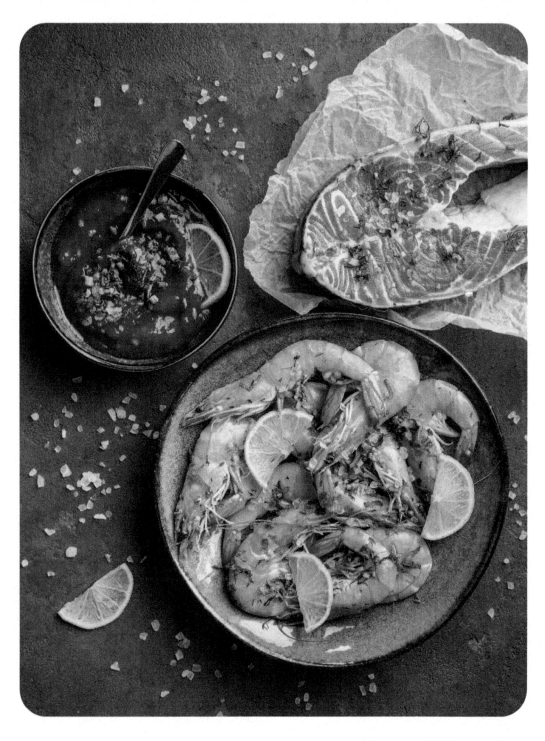

Spaghetti Squash Crab Blend

Prep time: 5 minutes | Cook time: 45 minutes | Serves 2

- 1 medium spaghetti squash
- 1 (6-ounce) package imitation crab meat (or 1 (6-ounce) can real lump crab meat)
- 1/2 teaspoon Old Bay seasoning, or to taste
- 1/4 teaspoon salt
- 1/8 teaspoon ground black pepper

Steps:
1. Preheat oven to 400°F.
2. Carefully cut squash in half lengthwise and place cut side up on a baking sheet. Bake until squash is tender, about 30–45 minutes depending on the size of the squash.
3. Peel squash away from skin with a fork and place strands in a medium bowl.
4. Add the crab meat and seasonings and mix well.

Per Serving
Calories: 82 | Fat: 1g | Protein: 15g | Sodium: 521mg | Fiber: 1g | Carbohydrates: 3g | Sugar: 2g

Shrimp Mexicana

Prep time: 8 minutes | Cook time: 5 minutes | Serves 4

- 6 egg whites
- ½ teaspoon the low sodium salt
- ¼ cup coconut flour
- ¼ cup almond milk
- ½ teaspoon cumin
- ¼ teaspoon chili powder
- 1 lime cut into wedges
- 1 tablespoon extra-virgin olive oil
- shredded lettuce for serving
- 1 teaspoon chili powder
- 1 teaspoon salt
- 1 lb. medium shrimp peeled and deveined
- 1 avocado pitted and diced
- fresh cilantro for serving

Steps:
1. Heat a skillet over medium heat, add the salt, chili pepper, and olive oil, and toss the shrimp in the mixture to coat. Place away.
2. Whisk the ingredients for the tortillas to make the batter.
3. Spray the skillet with almond oil spray before adding a thin coating of batter.
4. Cook for two minutes before turning over and cooking for an additional two minutes, or until faintly browned.
5. Serve shrimp, lettuce, avocado, and cilantro, on a tortilla.

Per Serving
Calories: 12|Fat: 0.3g | Saturated Fat: 0.1g | Carbohydrates: 0.5g | Protein: 1g

Langoustine and Red Pepper Rice-Free Paella

Prep time: 10 minutes | Cook time: 25 minutes | Serves 4

- 3 tbsp olive oil
- 2 red peppers, cut into cubes (about ½ cm thick)
- handful of black olives
- 1 zucchini (courgette) cut into cubes about ½ cm thick
- 1 tbsp paprika
- 7 large organic tomatoes cut into eight pieces
- 12oz langoustines - butterflied
- 1 fresh lemon, cut into quarters
- 1 serving of cooked fresh peas

Steps:
1. Heat oven to (150°C /300°f/Gas Mark 2).
2. Oil a baking tray and add the tomatoes, pepper, olives and zucchini.
3. Drizzle a little more olive oil over the vegetables and sprinkle salt and pepper and paprika over the top.
4. Oven bake for 30-40 minutes.
5. Whilst your vegetable mix is roasting, butterfly your langoustines:
6. Pull off the head and legs with your fingers and leave the tails for presentation.
7. Score down the centre of each prawn (do not slice in half) and then pull open on each side of the score to flatten.
8. Turn the oven up to (180°C /350°f/Gas Mark 4) and add your prawns to a roasting tray, drizzle with olive oil.
9. Cook for 6-7 minutes, ensuring piping hot before serving.
10. Serve the roasted vegetables (with added peas) in a pasta/rice dish with the prawns on top and the lemon wedges for squeezing.
11. Add salt and pepper to taste.

Per Serving
Calories: 353 | Protein: 40g | Carbs: 22g | Fat: 25g

Catch of the Day

Prep time: 10 minutes | Cook time: 25 minutes | Serves 4

- 1 whole trout cleaned and gutted (best caught yourself! if fishing doesn't come naturally, make sure it's sustainable)
- 2 green peppers, deseeded and chopped
- 8 cherry tomatoes halved
- handful of cilantro (coriander)
- handful of parsley
- 1 fresh lemon
- 1 clove minced garlic
- 1 tbsp olive oil,
- sprinkle of salt and pepper

Steps:

1. Heat oven to (190°C /375°f/Gas Mark 5).
2. Stuff the trout with the fresh herbs (save a handful for garnish), olive oil, and garlic.
3. Add to an oiled baking tray, surrounded by the vegetables.
4. Cook for 10-15 minutes – the fish must be piping hot before serving.
5. Serve with the lemon chunks and garnish with a handful of leftover herbs.

Per Serving

Calories: 504 | Protein: 36g | Carbs: 17g | Fat: 33g

Shrimp Stir-Fry

Prep time: 5 minutes | Cook time: 5 minutes | Serves 2

- 1 (16-ounce) bag frozen stir-fry vegetables
- 1 tablespoon olive oil
- 6 ounces shrimp, thawed
- 1/4 teaspoon minced garlic
- 1/4 teaspoon sea salt

Steps:

1. In a large pan over medium heat, cook vegetables with olive oil until thawed.
2. Add the rest of the ingredients, and cook until shrimp are fully cooked (they will turn opaque and pinkish), usually around 5 minutes.

Per Serving

Calories: 240 | Fat: 9g | Protein: 22g | Sodium: 486mg | Fiber: 6g | Carbohydrates: 20g | Sugar: 0g

Super Strong Salmon Frittata

Prep time: 10 minutes | Cook time: 25 minutes | Serves 4

- 2x 5oz wild salmon fillets
- 1 head of broccoli (pull off the florets)
- 1 tbsp olive oil
- handful of cilantro (coriander) and parsley
- 8 free range eggs, beaten
- 2 large peeled, sweet potatoes.

Steps:

1. Bring a pan of water to the boil on a high heat and add the sweet potatoes, cook for 20 minutes.
2. Steam the salmon over the pan for the last 15 minutes.
3. Add the broccoli in the same pan as the potatoes for the last 4-5 minutes of cooking and then drain.
4. Use your fork to flake the cooked salmon into a separate bowl whilst the potatoes and broccoli are cooling.
5. Use a knife to roughly chop the sweet potato into thin slices.
6. Mix the broccoli, sweet potato and salmon.
7. Heat the olive oil in a pan on a medium heat.
8. Add the potato and broccoli and salmon in a large omelette shape.
9. Mix eggs with herbs and pour over the ingredients.
10. Cook on a medium heat for 6-7 minutes (once edges are brown and a little crispy use a flat spatula to lift from the base of the pan and prevent sticking).
11. Continue to cook on a low heat for a further 5 minutes or until frittata can be easily lifted from the pan with your spatula.
12. Serve on a bed of salad!

Per Serving

Calories: 340 | Protein: 25g | Carbs: 15g | Fat: 20g

Training Thai Broth

Prep time: 10 minutes | Cook time: 25 minutes | Serves 4

- 2x 5oz skinless cod pieces
- 2 tbsp olive oil
- 1 tbsp coriander seeds
- 2 fresh limes
- 1 garlic clove
- 1 thumb size piece of minced ginger
- 1 white onion, chopped
- 1/4 cup spinach leaves
- handful of fresh basil leaves
- 1 pak choi
- 1 cup of homemade chicken stock
- 1 cup of good quality organic coconut milk (if available)
- 1 small green pepper deseeded and finely chopped
- 2 stems of spring onion, chopped

Steps:
1. Crush the fresh herbs and spices in a blender or use a pestle and mortar.
2. Mix in to 1 tbsp of olive oil until a paste is formed.
3. Heat a large pan or wok with sesame oil on a high heat.
4. Fry the onions, garlic and ginger until soft but not crispy or browned.
5. Add the spice paste with the coconut milk and stir.
6. Slowly add the stock until a broth is formed.
7. Now add your fish pieces and allow to simmer in the broth for 10-15 minutes.
8. Add the pak choi leaves 2-3 minutes before the end of the cooking time.
9. Plate and serve hot with the chilli and spring onion sprinkled over the top.

Per Serving
Calories: 440 | Protein: 40g | Carbs: 25g | Fat: 20g

Salmon and Sweet Potato Grain Bowls

Prep time: 15 minutes | Cook time: 30 minutes | Serves 4

- 4 tablespoons extra-virgin olive oil
- ½ teaspoon salt
- 4 salmon filets (4 ounces each), skinless
- 2 cups warm, cooked farro
- 2 tablespoons harissa
- 2 large sweet potatoes, peeled, cut into 1-inch cubes
- 4 cups baby spinach

Per Serving
Calories: 663 | Fat: 28 g | Carbohydrates: 62 g | Sugar: 8.9 g | Protein: 37 g

Steps:
1. Start by preheating the oven to 425°F. Grease a rimmed baking sheet with some cooking spray.
2. Add the harissa, olive oil, and salt into a bowl and mix well. Stir in the sweet potato cubes.
3. Spread the potatoes on the baking sheet and place them in the oven. Roast for 20 minutes.
4. Add the salmon into the bowl in which the sweet potatoes sat, and mix the salmon filets around in any harissa mixture in the bowl.
5. Place the fish and potatoes on the baking sheet, and roast until cooked.
6. In the meantime, combine the spinach and farro.
7. Distribute the farro mixture among four bowls. Distribute the sweet potatoes among the bowls. Place a salmon filet in each bowl and serve.

Super Human Mackerel & Brawny Beetroot

Prep time: 10 minutes | Cook time: 25 minutes | Serves 4

- 8oz skinned sweet potatoes
- 8oz smoked mackerel fillets, skin removed
- 4 spring onions, finely sliced
- 6oz small cooked beetroot, sliced into wedges
- small bunch dill, finely chopped
- 1 tsp caraway seeds
- 2 tbsp olive oil
- juice 1 lemon, zest of half

Steps:
1. Place a pan of water on a high heat and leave to boil.
2. Add the broccoli into the boiling water for 5-6 minutes.
3. Heat the oil in a separate pan on a medium heat and place the sea bass, skin down on to the pan. Hold the fillet for a few seconds to prevent the sides from curling up and shrinking.
4. Cook for 3 minutes and turn over.
5. Take the broccoli off the heat, drain and put to one side (check for taste first–crunchy is best but some like it softer!)
6. Cook the sea bass fillets for a further 2-3 minutes.
7. Add the lime juice to the sea bass and salt and pepper to taste.
8. Plate and serve the sea bass with the broccoli.

Per Serving
Calories: 223 | Protein: 20g | Carbs: 5g | Fat: 15g

Pasta with Tuna

Prep time: 10 minutes | Cook time: 30 minutes | Serves 2

- 4 ounces whole-wheat spaghetti
- 1 teaspoon grated lemon zest
- 1 tablespoon lemon juice or to taste
- ¼ teaspoon pepper
- ⅛ cup loosely packed fresh dill
- 1 ½ cups plus ⅛ cup water
- ¼ cup olives, pitted
- ¼ teaspoon salt or to taste
- 1 can (5 ounces) unsalted tuna, drained, flaked
- 1 tablespoon extra-virgin olive oil

Steps:
1. Add the spaghetti, lemon zest, salt, pepper, water, olives, and lemon juice into a pan and place it over high heat.
2. When the water starts boiling, turn down the heat and cook until the pasta is al dente and hardly any water remains in the pan.
3. Turn off the heat. Add the tuna, olive oil, and dill and mix well.
4. Serve.

Per Serving
Calories: 381 | Fat: 14.3 g | Carbohydrates: 41.2 g | Sugar: 2.2 g | Protein: 21 g

Calamari & Shrimp Paella

Prep time: 10 minutes | Cook time: 25 minutes | Serves 4

- 6 oz frozen cooked shrimp
- 1 cup calamari, fresh or frozen
- 1 tbsp olive oil
- 1 red onion, chopped
- 1 garlic clove, chopped
- 1 tsp paprika
- 1 tsp chili flakes
- 1 tbsp oregano
- 1 cup cooked brown rice
- 1/2 cup frozen peas

Steps:
1. Heat olive oil in a pan on a medium to high heat.
2. Add the onion and garlic and then fry for 2-3 minutes until soft.
3. Add the calamari and sauté for 5-10 minutes or until hot through.
4. Now add the shrimp and sauté for a further 5 minutes or until hot through.
5. Now add the herbs and spices, rice and frozen peas with 1/2 cup boiling water.
6. Stir until everything is warm and the water has been absorbed.
7. Plate up and serve.

Per Serving
Calories: 313 | Protein: 27g | Carbs: 33g | Fat: 11g

Salmon Burgers with Avocado

Prep time: 10 minutes | Cook time: 25 minutes | Serves 4

- 1 beaten free range egg
- 2 cans of wild salmon, drained
- 2 scallions, chopped
- 2 tbsp coconut oil
- 1 tsp dill, chopped
- 1 avocado
- 1 lime
- 1 cup cooked brown rice
- 1 cup spinach, washed

Steps:
1. Combine the salmon, egg, dill, scallions and 1 tbsp oil in a bowl, mixing well with your hands to form 2 patties.
2. Heat 1 tbsp oil over a medium heat in a skillet and cook the patties for 4 minutes each side until firm and browned.
3. Squeeze the lime juice over the top and flip once more.
4. Peel and slice the avocado.
5. Stack the burgers with the avocado sliced on top and a helping of spinach leaves and serve brown rice.

Per Serving
Calories: 611 | Protein: 62g | Carbs: 34g | Fat: 34g

Mighty Mussel Broth

Prep time: 10 minutes | Cook time: 25 minutes | Serves 4

- 10 oz mussels (without their shells) or 2 cups mussels with shells
- 1 white onion. finely diced
- 1 lemon, juiced
- 1 garlic clove, minced
- 1 stalk celery, sliced
- 1/2 cup veg stock
- 1/2 cup canned tomatoes
- 2 slices whole wheat bread
- 1 tsp olive oil

Steps:
1. Heat the oil in a large pot over a medium heat.
2. Add the onion, garlic and celery and sauté for 4-5 minutes or until starting to soften.
3. Add the tomatoes, stock and lemon juice and bring to the boil.
4. Turn down the heat and allow to simmer for 10 minutes.
5. Add the mussels and cook according to package directions (this will depend on whether they are in their shell or out).
6. The flesh should be vibrant and orange once cooked and the shells will be open.
7. Lightly toast the bread and serve on the side.
8. Dunk in and enjoy!

Per Serving
Calories: 447 | Protein: 40g | Carbs: 39g | Fat: 14g

Haddock & Kale Crumble

Prep time: 10 minutes | Cook time: 25 minutes | Serves 4

- 4x haddock fillets, skinless & boneless
- 2 cups curly kale
- 1/4 cup whole-wheat breadcrumbs
- 1/2 cup frozen peas
- 2 cups rice milk/whole milk
- 1/4 cup sesame seeds
- 1 tsp black pepper
- 1 tsp parsley

Steps:
1. Preheat oven to 400°f/200°c/Gas Mark 6.
2. Add the milk into a pan over a medium to high heat and bring to a simmer.
3. Add the haddock fillets, black pepper and parsley to the pan and lower the heat slightly.
4. Allow to simmer for 20-25 minutes or until cooked through.
5. Meanwhile, add the breadcrumbs and kale to a food processor and blitz together for 30 seconds (you still want a chunky texture).
6. Use a fork to flake the haddock fillets once cooked and return to the milk. Stir in the peas.
7. Into a deep oven dish, add the haddock and milk.
8. Top with the crispy kale mixture and bake in the oven for 25-30 minutes or until golden.

Per Serving
Calories: 620 | Protein: 66g | Carbs: 41g | Fat: 25g

Salmon Fettuccini

Prep time: 5 minutes |Cook time: 10 minutes |Serves 6

- 12 ounces fresh salmon fillets
- 12 ounces spelt fettuccini cooked
- 20 spinach leaves
- sea salt and pepper to taste
- 1 tablespoon clarified butter
- fresh basil
- 3 tablespoons lemon juice
- 2 cloves garlic pressed

Steps:
1. Fire up the barbecue.
2. Gently season the salmon with salt and pepper before grilling it for 6 minutes on each side.
3. Warm up the butter, lemon juice, and garlic to make the sauce.
4. Combine linguine, spinach, garlic-butter sauce, and fresh basil in a serving bowl.

Per Serving
Calories: 524| Fat: 12g| Sodium: 233mg| Carbohydrate: 76g| Protein: 35g

Chapter 9: Sides, and Salads

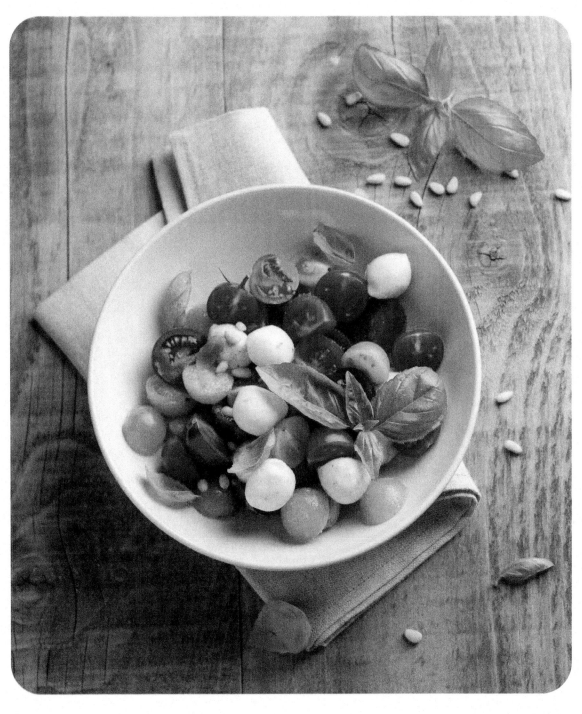

Spicy Peanut Tempeh Salad

Prep time: 5 minutes | Cook time: 4 minutes | Serves 4

- 6 ounces tempeh, cut into strips
- 3 cups chopped kale
- 2 tablespoons natural peanut butter
- 2 tablespoons white wine vinegar
- 4 tablespoons water
- Pinch ground cayenne pepper
- Pinch garlic powder

Steps:
1. In a large pan over medium heat, cook tempeh strips and kale about 3–4 minutes or until tempeh begins to look golden.
2. Add peanut butter, vinegar, water, cayenne, and garlic powder. Mix well until tempeh is coated with the mixture. Stir about 1 minute more and then serve.

Per Serving

Calories: 181 | Fat: 11g | Protein: 14g | Sodium: 59mg | Fiber: 2g | Carbohydrates: 12g | Sugar: 1g

Vegetarian Taco Salad

Prep time: 10 minutes | Cook time: 0 minute | Serves 4

For The Dressing:

- 4 tablespoons olive oil
- 4 teaspoons chili powder
- Juice of 2 limes
- 4 tablespoons tahini
- 1 teaspoon maple syrup or agave nectar

For The Salad:

- 2 cups chopped cherry tomatoes
- 1 cup cooked corn, fresh or frozen
- 8 cups Romaine lettuce or any greens of your choice
- 2 cups cooked or canned, drained black beans
- 1 avocado, peeled, pitted, diced

Steps:
1. To make the dressing: Add the olive oil, chili powder, lime juice, tahini, and maple syrup into a small bowl and whisk until smooth and well combined. Add a little water to dilute if necessary.
2. Combine the tomatoes, corn, lettuce, black beans, and avocado in a bowl. Drizzle the dressing over the salad. Toss well and serve.

Per Serving

Calories: 486.7 | Fat: 30.7 g | Carbohydrates: 45.9 g | Sugar: 4.5 g | Protein: 14.7 g

The Sweet Sailor Salad

Prep time: 5 minutes | Cook time: 23 to 28 minutes | Serves 4

- 1 cup raw spinach leaves
- 7oz lean grilled chopped turkey breast
- 1 tbsp grilled real bacon bits
- 2 eggs (free range)
- 4oz of chopped sweet potatoes
- 1 deseeded and sliced red, yellow and green pepper
- 1 avocado peeled and sliced (do this near to the end or it will start to turn brown)
- Sprinkle of salt and pepper

Steps:
1. Bring a pan of water to the boil on a high heat and add the chopped potatoes.
2. Cook for 15-20 minutes or according to packaging guidelines.
3. Combine the cooked meats with the spinach and peppers.
4. Drain the potatoes and leave to cool whilst placing a small pan of water to boil for the eggs.
5. Add the eggs once boiling and cook for 8 minutes for a medium-boiled and 10 minutes for a hard-boiled egg.
6. Run the eggs under a cold tap and peel.
7. Chop in half and add to your salad (here's where you can peel the avocado and add this).
8. Stir through your choice of olive oil, red/white wine vinegar and salt and pepper to taste.

Per Serving

Calories: 220 | Protein: 20g | Carbs: 13g | Fat: 10g

Muscle Building Steak & Balsamic Spinach Salad

Prep time: 5 minutes | Cook time: 8 minutes | Serves 2

- 8oz frying beef steak
- 1 chopped red onion
- 1 tsp of crushed garlic
- 1/4 cup baby spinach
- 1/4 cup watercress
- 4 cherry tomatoes, halved
- 2 tbsp of balsamic vinegar
- 2 tbsp olive oil
- Sprinkle of salt and pepper

Steps:
1. Sprinkle salt and pepper over steak.
2. Add a tbsp of olive oil to a griddle pan and heat on a high temperature.
3. Place the steak in the pan and cook for 8 minutes in total, turning the steak half way through.
4. Remove the steak from the pan and rest for 3 minutes.
5. Cut it into 2cm strips.
6. Get a bowl and add the chopped tomatoes, watercress, baby spinach, garlic and onions.
7. Place the steak strips in the bowl along with the vinegar and a tbsp of olive oil. Mix together.
8. Plate up and serve.

Per Serving
Calories: 308 | Protein: 34g | Carbs: 15g | Fat: 14g

Zucchini and Potato Bake

Prep time: 5 minutes |Cook time: 65 minutes| Serves 4

- 2 medium zucchini, sliced
- 4 medium potatoes, peeled and cut into large chunks
- 1 medium red bell pepper, seeded and chopped
- 1 clove garlic, minced
- $1/2$ cup bread crumbs
- $1/4$ cup olive oil
- 1 teaspoon paprika
- 1 teaspoon salt
- 1 teaspoon freshly ground black pepper

Steps:
1. Preheat oven to 400°F.
2. In a medium baking pan, toss all ingredients together, spreading evenly over the pan.
3. Bake 1 hour or until potatoes are tender, stirring occasionally.

Per Serving
Calories: 349.65 | Fat: 14.9 g | Protein: 7 g | Sodium: 710 mg | Fiber: 7.6 g | Carbohydrates: 48 g | Sugar: 7 g

Farro Salad

Prep time: 10 minutes | Cook time: 20 minutes | Serves 2

- 2 tablespoons lemon juice
- 1 ½ cups cooked farro
- ½ cup fresh mint leaves, torn
- 2 whole, canned artichoke hearts, rinsed, chopped
- ¼ cup chopped, salted, roasted pistachio nuts
- 3 tablespoons pomegranate seeds or dried cranberries
- 1 ½ ounces soft goat cheese, crumbled
- 2 tablespoons extra-virgin olive oil
- 3 cups packed baby arugula
- ¼ cup thinly sliced fresh basil leaves
- ¼ teaspoon salt or to taste

Steps:
1. Combine the farro, herbs, salt, artichoke, and arugula in a bowl.
2. Drizzle lemon juice and oil over the salad. Toss well.
3. Garnish with pomegranate, pistachios, and goat cheese, and serve.

Per Serving
Calories: 503 | Fat: 31 g | Carbohydrates: 29.7 g | Sugar: 26 g | Protein: 5.1 g

Shrimp Orzo Salad

Prep time: 5 minutes | Cook time: none | Serves 2

- 8 ounces orzo
- 1 pound shrimp, cooked, tails removed
- 1 cup cherry tomatoes, sliced in half
- 2 ounces reduced-fat feta cheese
- 1/4 cup chopped basil
- 1 tablespoon olive oil
- 1 tablespoon lemon juice
- 1/4 teaspoon salt
- 1/4 teaspoon ground black pepper

Steps:
1. Cook pasta according to package directions. Drain and rinse under cool water.
2. Combine shrimp, tomatoes, orzo, feta, basil, olive oil, and lemon juice in a large bowl.
3. Season with salt and pepper, mix well, and serve.

Per Serving

Calories: 461 | Fat: 11g | Protein: 57g | Sodium: 898mg | Fiber: 4g | Carbohydrates: 34g | Sugar: 4g

Spicy Roasted Spaghetti Squash

Prep time: 5 minutes | Cook time: 1 hour 7 minutes | Serves 4

- 1 (2-pound) spaghetti squash
- 2 tablespoons unsalted butter
- 1 shallot, minced
- 1 teaspoon salt
- 1/2 teaspoon freshly ground black pepper
- 1 teaspoon ground cayenne
- 1/2 teaspoon hot paprika
- 1/4 teaspoon allspice
- 1/4 teaspoon ground cloves

Steps:
1. Preheat oven to 400°F.
2. Pierce squash with point of a knife multiple times. Place on a baking sheet. Roast 1 hour or until squash is easily pierced with a fork.
3. Halve the squash. Remove seeds and discard. Scoop out the flesh. Shred with a fork. Set aside.
4. Melt butter in a skillet. Add shallot and sauté 2 minutes. Add squash and spices. Sauté an additional 5 minutes. Serve immediately.

Per Serving

Calories: 71 | Fat: 6g | Protein: 1g | Sodium: 594mg | Fiber: 0g | Carbohydrates: 5g | Sugar: 0g

Broiled Tomato Sandwich

Prep time: 5 minutes |Cook time: 65 minutes| Serves 2

- 2 tablespoons olive oil
- 2 tablespoons balsamic vinegar
- 1 large tomato, sliced
- 3 tablespoons reduced-fat mayonnaise
- $^1/_2$ teaspoon dried parsley
- $^1/_4$ teaspoon dried oregano
- $^1/_4$ teaspoon freshly ground black pepper
- 3 tablespoons grated vegetarian Parmesan cheese, divided
- 4 slices sprouted or whole-grain bread, lightly toasted

Steps:
1. Preheat oven to broil.
2. Add olive oil and vinegar to a small bowl and whisk well.
3. Add tomatoes, cover, and marinate 30–60 minutes.
4. In a separate small bowl, mix mayonnaise, parsley, oregano, pepper, and 2 teaspoons Parmesan.
5. Place bread slices on a baking sheet and evenly spread mayonnaise mixture over each slice, topping 2 of the slices with the marinated tomatoes. Place remaining 2 bread slices on top of tomatoes, mayonnaise side down.
6. Broil 5 minutes or until cheese turns golden brown. Serve immediately.

Per Serving

Calories: 339 | Fat: 32 g | Protein: 4.7 g | Sodium: 270 mg | Fiber: 1.2 g | Carbohydrates: 7.5 g | Sugar: 4.9 g

Chickpea Salad

Prep time: 5 minutes |Cook time: 5 minutes| Serves 4

- 1 (19-ounce) can chickpeas, drained and rinsed
- 1 stalk celery, chopped
- $^1/_2$ medium onion, peeled and chopped
- 1 tablespoon mayonnaise
- 1 tablespoon lemon juice
- 1 teaspoon dried dill

Steps:
1. In a medium bowl mash chickpeas with a fork.
2. Add all other ingredients, mix well, and refrigerate until ready to eat.

Per Serving
Calories: 125 | Fat: 4.2 g | Protein: 5.2 g | Sodium: 33 mg | Fiber: 4.7 g | Carbohydrates: 17.4 g | Sugar: 3.5 g

Protein Packed Egg & Bean Salad

Prep time: 5 minutes | Cook time: none | Serves 8

- 16oz of cooked black beans, drained & rinsed
- 16oz of cooked cannellini beans, drained & rinsed
- 16oz of cooked kidney beans, drained & rinsed
- 6 hard-boiled eggs, sliced
- 1 celery stick chopped
- ½ Onion, chopped
- Handful of olives, sliced
- 3 tsp of hot pepper sauce
- ½ Tsp of salt
- ¼ Tsp of pepper
- 3 tsp of italian salad dressing

Steps:
1. Drain the beans, then rinse, and finally drain again.
2. Combine celery, olives, onions, salad dressing, seasonings, and beans. Carefully mix. Refrigerate for at least 2 hours, preferably overnight.
3. When ready to serve. Drain off the salad dressing first, then add eggs.
4. Carefully mix so as not to mash the beans.
5. Serve.

Per Serving
Calories: 366 | Protein: 15g | Carbs: 30g | Fat: 14g

Baked Eggplant and Bell Pepper

Prep time: 5 minutes | Cook time: 30 minutes | Serves 2

- 1 medium eggplant, sliced
- 1 medium green bell pepper, seeded and diced
- 2 celery stalks, sliced
- 2 cloves garlic, minced
- 1 teaspoon dried oregano
- 1/4 teaspoon salt
- 1/8 teaspoon ground black pepper
- 1/4 cup red wine vinegar

Steps:
1. Preheat oven to 400°F.
2. Place eggplant, green pepper, and celery in a 13" × 9" glass dish.
3. Sprinkle with minced garlic, oregano, salt, and black pepper.
4. Pour red wine vinegar over the top.
5. Cover dish with aluminum foil and bake 30 minutes.

Per Serving
Calories: 85 | Fat: 1g | Protein: 3g | Sodium: 336mg | Fiber: 10g | Carbohydrates: 19g | Sugar: 8g

Chapter 10: Pasta and Soups

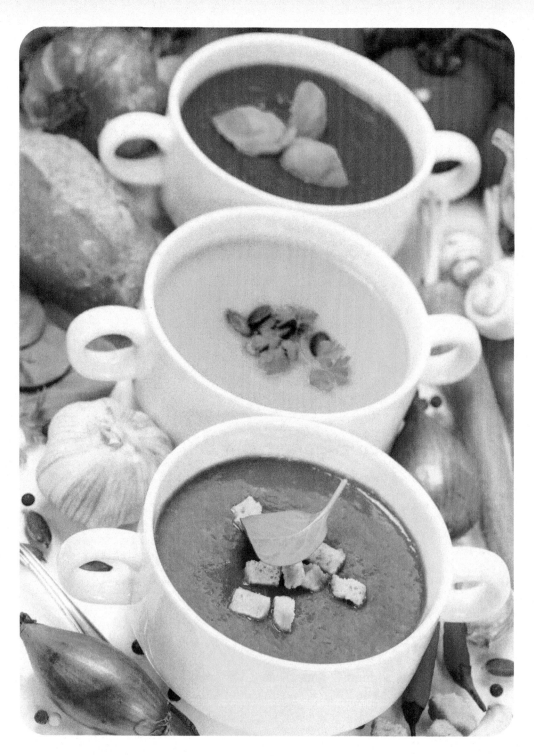

Farfalle with Chicken and Pesto

Prep time: 5 minutes | Cook time: 8 minutes | Serves 4

- 8 ounces farfalle
- 1/2 pound fresh green beans, ends trimmed
- 1/2 cup reserved pasta water
- 1/2 cup reduced-fat pesto sauce
- 2 cups bite-sized pieces grilled chicken

Steps:
1. Cook pasta according to package directions. Drain and reserve 1/2 cup pasta water.
2. Place green beans in a shallow pan with enough fresh water to cover them. Cover and steam over medium heat 8 minutes. Drain.
3. Combine cooked pasta, pesto, reserved pasta water, chicken, and green beans in a large bowl and stir to combine.

Per Serving

Calories: 308 | Fat: 10g | Protein: 27g | Sodium: 421mg | Fiber: 5g | Carbohydrates: 51g | Sugar: 6g

Vegetable and Tortilla Soup

Prep time: 5 minutes | Cook time: 35 minutes | Serves 12

- 2 tablespoons vegetable oil
- 1 (16-ounce) package frozen stir-fry mix
- 2 cloves garlic, minced
- 3 tablespoons ground cumin
- 1 (28-ounce) can crushed tomatoes
- 3 (4-ounce) cans chopped green chile peppers, drained
- 4 (14-ounce) cans vegetable broth
- 1 (11-ounce) can whole kernel corn
- 12 ounces whole-grain tortilla chips

Steps:
1. Heat oil in a large saucepan over medium heat. Add stir-fry, garlic, and cumin and cook 5 minutes, stirring frequently. Add tomatoes, peppers, and broth.
2. Bring soup to a boil, then reduce to a simmer and continue cooking 30 minutes.
3. Mix corn into soup and cook an additional 5 minutes.
4. Fill each bowl halfway with tortilla chips, top with soup, and serve.

Per Serving

Calories: 137 | Fat: 3.87 g | Protein: 3.6 g | Sodium: 499 mg | Fiber: 3.5 g | Carbohydrates: 24.85 g | Sugar: 5 g

Garlic Cheddar Cauliflower Soup

Prep time: 5 minutes | Cook time: 10 minutes | Serves 2

- 2 tablespoons olive oil
- 1 small yellow onion, peeled and chopped
- 2 cloves garlic, peeled and minced
- 1 medium head cauliflower, cored, outer leaves removed, and chopped
- 4 cups low-sodium chicken broth
- ½ cup shredded sharp cheddar cheese
- ¼ cup grated parmesan cheese

Steps:
1. Heat oil in a large saucepan over medium heat. Sauté onion and garlic 5 minutes.
2. Add cauliflower and broth. Increase heat to high and bring to a boil.
3. Reduce heat to medium-low and simmer 20 minutes until cauliflower is soft.
4. Remove from heat, then transfer soup to a blender and process until smooth (or use a handheld blender).
5. Return soup to pot, stir in Cheddar and Parmesan, and heat, stirring constantly, over medium heat 5 minutes until cheeses melt. Serve hot.

Per Serving

Calories: 351 | Fat: 23g | Sodium: 485mg | Carbohydrates: 18g | Fiber: 7g | Sugar: 8g | Protein: 18g

Broccoli and "Cheese" Soup

Prep time: 5 minutes | Cook time: 10 minutes | Serves 4

- 1 teaspoon olive oil
- 1 medium yellow onion, peeled and chopped
- 2 teaspoons minced garlic
- 3 cups low-sodium chicken broth
- 1 cup full-fat coconut milk
- 5 cups roughly chopped broccoli florets
- $1/3$ cup nutritional yeast
- $1/4$ teaspoon salt

Steps:
1. Heat oil in a large pot over medium heat. Add onion and garlic and sauté for 3–4 minutes until softened.
2. Add chicken broth, coconut milk, broccoli, nutritional yeast, and salt. Stir to combine.
3. Reduce heat to medium-low and simmer for 12–15 minutes until broccoli is tender.
4. Remove from heat, then transfer soup to a blender and process until smooth or until desired consistency is reached (or use a handheld blender). Serve immediately.

Per Serving
Calories: 208 | Fat: 17g | Sodium: 178mg | Carbohydrates: 11g | Fiber: 1g | Sugar: 6g | Protein: 3g

Bean and Leek Soup

Prep time: 5 minutes | Cook time: 5 minutes | Serves 4

- 2 teaspoons olive oil
- 4 medium leeks (bulb only), chopped
- 2 cloves garlic, chopped
- 2 cups low-sodium vegetable broth
- 2 (16-ounce) cans cannellini beans, drained and rinsed
- 2 bay leaves
- 2 teaspoons ground cumin
- $1/2$ cup whole-wheat couscous

Steps:
1. Heat olive oil in a large saucepan over medium heat. Add leeks and garlic and sauté until tender.
2. Add broth, beans, bay leaves, and cumin and bring to a boil.
3. Reduce to a simmer, stir in couscous, and simmer, covered, 5 minutes.
4. Remove bay leaves and serve warm.

Per Serving
Calories: 301 | Fat: 3.9 g | Protein: 14.72 g | Sodium: 142 mg | Fiber: 13 g | Carbohydrates: 51 g | Sugar: 5 g

Light Fettuccine Alfredo

Prep time: 5 minutes | Cook time: 15 minutes | Serves 2

- 12 ounces dry fettuccine
- $2 1/2$ teaspoons salt, divided
- 1 head broccoli, cut into florets, stalk peeled and sliced
- $1 1/2$ cups skim milk
- 1 tablespoon unsalted butter
- 1 tablespoon flour
- $3/4$ cup freshly grated Parmesan cheese, plus more for serving

Steps:
1. Cook pasta according to package directions. Drain.
2. Bring a pot of water with 1 teaspoon salt to a boil and cook broccoli 3 minutes until tender.
3. Heat milk and butter in a large saucepan over low heat and slowly whisk in flour until thickened.
4. Remove from heat and stir in Parmesan and remaining salt. Add pasta and broccoli and cook, stirring over low heat until heated through, about 3–5 minutes.

Per Serving
Calories: 958 | Fat: 21 g | Protein: 46 g | Sodium: 1,278 mg | Fiber: 8 g | Carbohydrates: 144 g | Sugar: 16 g

Lemon, Herb, and Cheese Pasta

Prep time: 5 minutes |Cook time: 5 minutes| Serves 4

- 1 (16-ounce) package penne
- $^1/_2$ cup reserved pasta water
- 2 tablespoons butter
- 1 cup ricotta cheese
- Zest of 1 medium lemon
- $^3/_4$ teaspoon salt
- $^1/_4$ teaspoon freshly ground black pepper

Steps:
1. Cook pasta according to package directions and drain, reserving 1/2 cup pasta water. Return pasta to the pot.
2. In a medium bowl, whisk together pasta water, butter, and ricotta until a rich, creamy sauce forms.
3. Pour sauce over hot pasta. Add zest, salt, and pepper and toss.

Per Serving
Calories: 579 | Fat: 16 g | Protein: 22 g | Sodium: 496 mg | Fiber: 4 g | Carbohydrates: 87 g | Sugar: 4 g

Artichoke and Olive Pasta

Prep time: 5 minutes | Cook time: 10 minutes | Serves 4

- 2 tablespoons olive oil
- 3 cloves garlic, minced
- 2 shallots, minced
- 10 ounces frozen artichoke hearts, defrosted
- 1 cup halved large, oil-cured green olives
- 1/2 cup toasted fresh bread crumbs
- 1/3 cup grated Parmesan cheese
- 1/4 cup chopped fresh Italian parsley
- 10 ounces hot cooked fresh linguine

Steps:
1. In a saucepan, heat the oil over medium heat. Add the garlic and shallots and cook until fragrant, about 3–5 minutes.
2. Add the artichoke hearts and olives. Cook until the artichokes are cooked through, about 5 minutes.
3. Remove from heat and stir in the remaining ingredients. Serve immediately.

Per Serving
Calories: 507 | Fat: 14g | Protein: 17g | Sodium: 546mg | Fiber: 8g | Carbohydrates: 82g | Sugar: 3g

Asian Shrimp Noodles

Prep time: 10 minutes |Cook time: 15 minutes| Serves 2

- 1 (16-ounce) package dry rice noodles
- 1 bunch green onions
- 1 tablespoon finely chopped fresh ginger
- 3 tablespoons olive oil
- 1 pound shrimp, peeled and deveined
- 1 teaspoon salt
- 1 teaspoon freshly ground black pepper
- $^3/_4$ cup water
- $^1/_3$ cup soy sauce
- 2 (12-ounce) bags shredded cabbage mix for coleslaw

Steps:
1. Cook noodles according to package directions and drain, rinsing under cold water.
2. In a large skillet over medium heat, sauté green onions and ginger with olive oil 2 minutes.
3. Add shrimp to skillet in single layer with salt and pepper. Cook 3–4 minutes or until shrimp just turn opaque, stirring frequently. Remove shrimp and set aside.
4. Add water and soy sauce to the same skillet, scraping up browned bits. Stir in cabbage mix and cover and cook 6 minutes over medium heat, stirring often.
5. Transfer cabbage and shrimp mix to a bowl with noodles, mixing well before serving.

Per Serving
Calories: 1,193 | Fat: 24 g | Protein: 48 g | Sodium: 5,192 mg | Fiber: 5 g | Carbohydrates: 187 g | Sugar: 2 g

Taco Corn Chowder

Prep time: 5 minutes | Cook time: 10 minutes | Serves 4

- 2 tablespoons olive oil
- 8 cups frozen corn kernels, thawed
- 1 medium yellow onion, peeled and diced
- 1 tablespoon taco seasoning
- 1 teaspoon salt
- 6 cups low-sodium chicken broth
- ½ cup shredded pepper jack cheese

Steps:

1. In a large pot over medium-high heat, heat oil. Add corn, onion, taco seasoning, and salt.
2. Sauté for 7–8 minutes until onion is soft.
3. Remove one-third of the mixture and set aside.
4. Add broth to the pot and bring to a boil. Reduce heat to medium-low and simmer for 15 minutes.
5. Remove from heat, then transfer soup to a blender and process until smooth (or use a handheld blender).
6. Return soup to pot and stir in the reserved corn mixture. Simmer over medium-low heat for 3 minutes.
7. Ladle soup into four bowls and top with cheese. Serve immediately.

Per Serving

Calories: 412 | Fat: 12g | Sodium: 857mg | Carbohydrates: 67g | Fiber: 4g | Sugar: 12g | Protein: 13g

Sweet Potato Soup

Prep time: 5 minutes | Cook time: 10 minutes | Serves 4

- 6 large sweet potatoes, peeled and chopped
- 1 large onion, peeled and chopped
- 3 stalks celery, chopped
- 2 teaspoons poultry seasoning
- 4 cups low-sodium chicken broth
- 2 cups milk

Steps:

1. Add sweet potatoes, onion, celery, and poultry seasoning to a large pot. Add broth and top off with water until vegetables are just covered.
2. Bring to a boil over high heat. Reduce heat to medium-low and simmer 10–15 minutes until vegetables are tender.
3. Remove from heat, then transfer soup to a blender and process until smooth (or use a handheld blender). Return soup to pot and stir in milk. Heat over medium-low heat for 5 minutes. Serve hot.

Per Serving

Calories: 178 | Fat: 3g | Sodium: 121mg | Carbohydrates: 29g | Fiber: 4g | Sugar: 12g | Protein: 8g

Slow Cooker Black Bean Soup

Prep time: 5 minutes | Cook time: 10 minutes | Serves 6

- 2 tablespoons olive oil
- 2 medium carrots, peeled and chopped
- 2 stalks celery, chopped
- 1 medium onion, peeled and chopped
- ¼ cup tomato paste
- 3 cloves garlic, peeled and minced
- 1 ½ teaspoons ground cumin
- 3 (15-ounce) cans black beans, drained and rinsed
- 1 cup frozen or canned corn
- 3 cups vegetable broth

Steps:

1. Heat oil in a medium skillet over medium-high heat.
2. Add carrots, celery, and onion to the pan and sauté 5 minutes until slightly softened.
3. Stir in tomato paste, garlic, and cumin and continue to cook 2 minutes, stirring frequently.
4. Transfer mixture to a 4- to 6-quart slow cooker. Stir in beans, corn, and broth. Cook on high for 4 hours.
5. Serve warm or allow to cool and refrigerate for up to 5 days.

Per Serving

Calories: 392 | Fat: 6g | Sodium: 102mg | Carbohydrates: 66g | Fiber: 2g | Sugar: 6g | Protein: 18g

Chapter 11: Sauces, Dressings, and Rubs

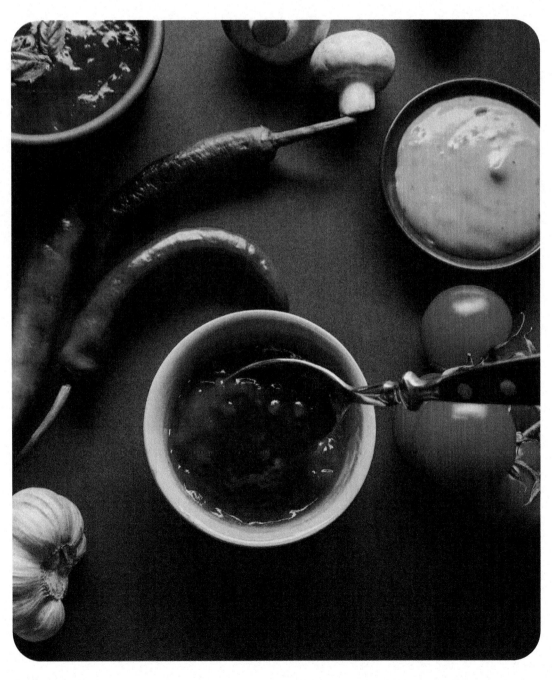

Sun-Dried Tomato Vinaigrette

Prep time: 5 minutes | Cook time: none | Serves 2

- 1/3 cup sun-dried tomatoes
- 1/4 cup red wine vinegar
- 1 tablespoon olive oil
- 1 clove garlic, minced

Steps:

1. Blend all ingredients in blender or food processor until smooth.

Per Serving

Calories: 90 | Fat: 7g | Protein: 1g | Sodium: 191mg | Fiber: 1g | Carbohydrates: 5g | Sugar: 3g

Dijon Vinaigrette

Prep time: 10 minutes | Cook time: 15 minutes | Serves 2

- 2 tbsps. red wine vinegar
- 1 tsp. Dijon mustard
- ½ tsp. honey

Steps:

1. Mix all the directions in a bowl and stir to reach proper consistency.
2. Serve and enjoy!

Per Serving

Calories: 21 | Fat: 0g | Carbohydrates: 3g

Macro Caesar Dressing

Prep time: 10 minutes | Cook time: 15 minutes | Serves 15

- 1 egg yolk
- 2 tsps. Dijon mustard
- 1 tbsp. anchovy paste
- 2 tbsps. lemon juice
- 2 cloves garlic
- 1 tbsp. oregano
- 1 tsp. salt
- 1 tsp. black pepper
- ½ cup of olive oil
- ½ cup parmesan cheese

Steps:

1. Place all thedirections in a blender except the olive oil and pulse until smooth.
2. Pulse in the olive oil to achieve a thick consistency.
3. Serve over a salad and enjoy!

Per Serving

Calories: 114 | Fat: 7g | Carbohydrates: 1g | Protein: 2g

Macro Blue Cheese Dressing

Prep time: 10 minutes | Cook time: 15 minutes | Serves 16

- 1 cup mayonnaise
- ½ cup sour cream
- 4 oz. blue cheese crumbles
- 1 tsp. lemon juice
- ¼ cup unsweetened almond milk (or any milk of choice)
- ½ tsp. sea salt (to taste)
- ¼ tsp. black pepper (to taste)

Steps:

1. Stir all directions in a bowl, crushing the blue cheese crumbles to incorporate their flavor.
2. Serve in a salad and enjoy!

Per Serving

Calories: 99 | Fat: 1/2g | Carbohydrates: 4g | Protein: 6g

Basil Vinaigrette

Prep time: 10 minutes | Cook time: 15 minutes | Serves 4

- ⅓ cup champagne wine vinegar can use red wine vinegar or white balsamic vinegar
- ½ clove garlic
- ¼ cup fresh parsley
- ¾ cup fresh basil
- ¾ cup lemon juice
- ¼ tsp. kosher salt
- ¼ tsp. fresh ground pepper
- 2 tbsps. honey
- 1 tbsp. olive oil
- 100gnon-fat Greek yogurt

Steps:
1. Blend all of the directions except the yogurt and olive oil in a blender until smooth, drizzling in olive oil as it blends.
2. Add the yogurt and blend until smooth.
3. Serve over a salad and enjoy!

Per Serving
Calories: 63 | Fat: 7g | Carbohydrates: 3g | Protein: 9g

Macro Thousand Island Dressing

Prep time: 10 minutes | Cook time: 15 minutes | Serves 12

- 1 cup mayonnaise
- ¼ cup sugar-free ketchup
- 2 tbsps. apple cider vinegar
- 2 tbsps. no sugar added sweetener
- 1 ½ tbsps. dill pickles (finely chopped)
- 2 tsps. white onion (minced)
- ¼ tsp. sea salt
- ⅛ tsp. black pepper

Steps:
1. Mix together all directions in a bowl, stirring to reach dressing consistency.
2. Serve in a salad and enjoy!

Per Serving
Calories: 87 | Fat: 5g | Carbohydrates: 7g | Protein: 5g

Dry Rub For Ribs

Prep time: 5 minutes | Cook time: none | Serves 1

- 3 tablespoons brown sugar
- 11/2 tablespoons paprika
- 11/2 tablespoons salt
- 11/2 tablespoons ground black pepper
- 1 teaspoon garlic powder

Steps:
1. In a small bowl, mix all ingredients together.
2. Use immediately or store until ready for the ribs.

Per Serving
Calories: 220 | Fat: 2g | Protein: 3g | Sodium: 3,450mg | Fiber: 7g | Carbohydrates: 54g | Sugar: 41g

Lemon Tahini Dressing

Prep time: 5 minutes | Cook time: 10 minutes | Makes ½ Cup

- ¼ cup tahini
- ¼ cup lemon juice
- 1 tablespoon maple syrup or agave nectar

Steps:
In a small bowl, whisk all ingredients together. Use immediately or refrigerate for up to 3 days.

Per Serving
Calories: 114 | Fat: 9g | Sodium: 0mg | Carbohydrates: 4g | Fiber: 0g | Sugar: 4g | Protein: 4g

Easy Peanut Sauce

Prep time: 5 minutes | Cook time: 10 minutes | Makes ½ Cup

- ½ cup powdered peanut butter
- ½ cup low-sodium soy sauce or coconut aminos
- 4 teaspoons ground ginger

Steps:
1. Combine all ingredients in a small bowl and mix well.
2. Serve immediately or refrigerate, covered, for up to 5 days.

Per Serving

Calories: 130 | Fat: 4g | Sodium: 1,536mg | Carbohydrates: 12g | Fiber: 2g | Sugar: 4g | Protein: 12g

Macro Ranch Dressing

Prep time: 10 minutes | Cook time: 15 minutes | Serves 16

- 1 tbsp. dried parsley
- 2 tsps. garlic powder
- 2 tsps. onion powder
- ¼ tsp. ground black pepper
- ½ tsp. salt
- 1 tbsp. fresh chives
- 1 cup nonfat plain Greek yogurt
- ¾ cup buttermilk
- 1 tsp. Dijon mustard
- 1 tsp. lemon juice

Steps:
1. Pulse the parsley and chives in a blender until they reach a flake shape.
2. Using a spatula, put the herbs on the sides of the bowl down to avoid them sticking to the sides.
3. Add all remaining directions to the blender and pulse until fully incorporated, using the spatula to reincorporate the herbs if necessary.
4. Serve over a salad and enjoy!

Per Serving

Calories: 87 | Fat: 5g | Carbohydrates: 7g | Protein: 5g

Kale Slaw & Creamy Dressing

Prep time: 5 minutes | Cook time: 5 minutes | Serves 2

- $^1/_3$ cup sesame seeds
- 1 bell pepper
- $^1/_3$ cup sunflower seeds
- 1 red onion
- 1 bunch of kale
- 4 cups of red cabbage shredded
- 1 piece of root ginger
- fresh coriander
- 1 serving of cashew dressing

Steps:
Toss all the ingredients together.

Per Serving

Calories: 97 | Carbs: 5.7g | Fat: 6.8g | Protein: 1.7g

Classic Vinaigrette

Prep time: 10 minutes | Cook time: 15 minutes | Serves 2

- 2 tbsps. red wine vinegar
- 2 tbsps. olive oil
- salt and pepper to taste

Steps:
1. Whisk the oil and vinegar in a cup until mixed to proper consistency.
2. Serve over a salad and add salt and pepper to taste. Enjoy!

Per Serving

Calories: 123 | Fat: 14g | Carbohydrates: 1g | Protein: 0g

Chapter 12: Holidays

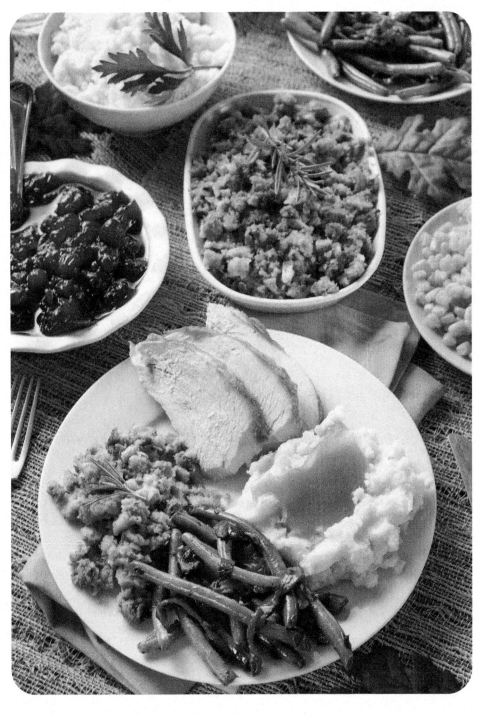

Spice-Rubbed Roasted Turkey Breast

Prep time: 5 minutes | Cook time: 2 hour 30 minutes | Serves 8

- 1 (5-pound) turkey breast
- 2 teaspoons garlic powder
- 2 teaspoons onion powder
- 1 teaspoon cayenne
- 1 teaspoon all-natural sea salt
- 1 teaspoon freshly ground black pepper
- 1 tablespoon olive oil
- 1 large lemon, sliced

Steps:
1. Preheat oven to 325°F, and prepare a roasting pan with olive oil spray. Set turkey breast in roasting pan (if previously frozen, make sure it is thawed).
2. Combine all spices in a small mixing bowl, and mix well.
3. Coat turkey breast with olive oil, and sprinkle spice mixture over turkey breast. Top with lemon slices.
4. Cook turkey breast 11/2–21/2 hours, or until internal temperature reads 165–170°F. Slice and serve hot.

Per Serving
Calories: 331 | Fat: 4g | Protein: 69g | Sodium: 433mg | Fiber: 1g | Carbohydrates: 2g | Sugar: 0g

Egg Roll in a Bowl

Prep time: 10 minutes | Cook time: 20 minutes | Serves 2-4

- 1 lb. (450g) ground pork
- 1 tbsp. (15ml) olive oil
- 1 small onion, diced
- 3 garlic cloves, minced
- 1 tsp. (5g) ground ginger
- 1/2 tsp. (2.5g) ground black pepper
- 1/4 tsp. (1g) salt
- 1/4 tsp. (1g) red pepper flakes (optional)
- 4 c. (400g) coleslaw mix (shredded cabbage and carrots)
- 1/4 c. (60ml) soy sauce (or tamari for gluten-free)
- 2 tbsp. (30ml) rice vinegar
- 2 green onions, thinly sliced
- 1 tbsp. (15ml) sesame oil

Steps:
1. Heat up the olive oil in a large skillet over medium-high heat. Put the ground pork in the skillet and cook it until it is browned, while breaking it up into small crumbles.
2. Add the diced onion and minced garlic to the skillet and cook for 2-3 minutes, or until the onion has become translucent.
3. Add the ground ginger, black pepper, salt, and red pepper flakes (if using) to the skillet and stir to combine.
4. Put the coleslaw mix into the skillet and stir it with the pork and onion mixture. Cook for 3-4 minutes, or until the vegetables have slightly softened.
5. In a separate small bowl, mix the soy sauce, rice vinegar, and sesame oil together using a whisk. Pour the sauce onto the skillet mixture and stir until everything is mixed.
6. Cook for an additional 2-3 minutes or until the vegetables are tender and the sauce is heated through.
7. Take the skillet off the heat and sprinkle thinly sliced green onions over the top.
8. Serve the dish hot and enjoy!

Per Serving
Calories: 360 | Fat: 25g | Carbohydrates: 8g | Fiber: 3g | Protein: 25g

Super Steak with Spicy Rice & Beans

Prep time: 5 minutes | Cook time: 12 minutes | Serves 2

- 2 12oz sirloin steaks
- 4 tsp olive oil
- 1 small onion, sliced
- 1 cup brown long-grain rice
- 1½tsp fajita seasoning
- 1 can of drained kidney beans
- Handful of chopped coriander leaves
- 2 tbsp tomato salsa, to serve

Steps:
1. Pour 3 tsp of oil into a deep saucepan on a medium heat and add the onion. Fry the onion for around 4 minutes.
2. Then add ½ the fajita seasoning and long grain rice. Cook for 1 minute. Add 300ml of boiling water to the saucepan and stir in. Cover the saucepan and let simmer for 20 minutes until the water has been absorbed and the rice is fluffy. Add the kidney beans and keep the pan warm.
3. While the rice is cooking, sprinkle salt and pepper over the steak as well as ½ fajita seasoning. Pre-heat a griddle pan on a high heat, add the steaks and cook for 8 minutes in total, turning the steaks half way through.
4. Add the rice to a bowl and mix in the coriander. Add a tbsp of tomato salsa to each of the steaks and serve.

Per Serving
Calories:650 | Protein: 48g | Carbs: 60g | Fat: 26g

Muscle Mint Lamb Steaks

Prep time: 5 minutes | Cook time: 34 minutes | Serves 2

- 4 8oz lamb leg steaks
- 2 tbsp olive oil
- 2 chopped garlic cloves
- 1 tbsp balsamic vinegar
- Handful of chopped mint leaves

Steps:

1. Get a bowl and add the mint, vinegar and garlic and mix together.
2. Add the lamb to the bowl and leave to marinade for at least 30 minutes.
3. Pre-heat a griddle pan on a medium to high heat and cook the lamb for 4 minutes each side or until cooked through.
4. Serve alone or with your choice of salad for a delicious accompaniment.

Per Serving

Calories:367 | Protein: 41g | Carbs: 2g | Fat: 22g

Super Lamb Steaks with Mediterranean Veg

Prep time: 5 minutes | Cook time: 4 minutes | Serves 2

- 2 8oz lamb leg/breast steaks
- 2 chopped courgettes
- 2 tbsp olive oil
- Handful of rocket
- 2 garlic cloves, chopped
- 8 halved baby cherry tomatoes
- Handful of chopped coriander

Steps:

1. Preheat the grill.
2. Add the oil to a pan and heat on a medium heat.
3. Throw in the courgettes, tomatoes and garlic and fry until courgettes and tomatoes are soft.
4. Add the rocket and coriander and stir in.
5. Meanwhile, sprinkle some salt and pepper over the lamb steaks. Place the lamb on a tray and grill for 4 minutes. each side.
6. Serve alongside the veg.

Per Serving

Calories:308 | Protein: 34g | Carbs: 15g | Fat: 14g

Pork Loin with Baked Apples

Prep time: 5 minutes | Cook time: 50 minutes | Serves 4

- 1/4 cup unsweetened applesauce
- 2 tablespoons filtered water
- 3 medium gala apples, cored, peeled, and cut into slices
- 1 teaspoon cinnamon
- 1 pound pork tenderloin
- 1 teaspoon all-natural sea salt
- 1 tablespoon agave nectar

Steps:

1. Preheat oven to 400°F and spray a 13" × 9" pan with olive oil spray.
2. Mix applesauce, water, and apples in a mixing bowl with cinnamon.
3. Layer apples evenly in the pan, and cook 20 minutes, or until slightly softened.
4. Place pork tenderloin in the middle of the pan and surround with apples.
5. Sprinkle tenderloin with sea salt, and drizzle agave nectar over the pork and the apples.
6. Return pan to oven for another 30 minutes, or until the internal temperature reads 165°F.

Per Serving

Calories: 204 | Fat: 3g | Protein: 24g | Sodium: 650mg | Fiber: 2g | Carbohydrates: 22g | Sugar: 18g

Brawn Bison Burger

Prep time: 5 minutes | Cook time: 12 to 15 minutes | Serves 2

- 18oz of ground organic bison
- 3 chopped jalapeno peppers
- ½ Chopped red onion
- 1 finely chopped shallot
- 1 egg (free range)
- 2 crushed garlic cloves
- Sprinkle of salt and pepper

Steps:

1. Pre-heat grill to a medium heat.
2. Cover a baking tray with foil.
3. Mix all of the ingredients together in a large bowl and form palm sized patties with your hands.
4. Place your bison patties in the middle of the baking tray and slot under the grill.
5. Grill patties for around 12 – 15 minutes, turning them over halfway through.
6. Take patties out of the grill when both sides are golden and the meat is cooked through.
7. Plate and serve with a side salad.

Per Serving

Calories:292 | Protein: 43g | Carbs: 7g | Fat: 23g

Cauliflower Fried Rice

Prep time: 10 minutes | Cook time: 20 minutes | Serves 2-4

- 1 medium head of cauliflower (about 4 C. riced)
- 1 tbsp. (15ml) olive oil
- 1 small onion, diced
- 2 garlic cloves, minced
- 1 medium carrot, diced
- 1/2 C. (75g) frozen peas
- 2 large eggs, lightly beaten
- 2 tbsp. (30ml) soy sauce (use tamari for gluten-free or coconut aminos for paleo)
- salt and black pepper, to taste

Optional Toppings:

- sliced green onions, sesame seeds, hot sauce

Steps:

1. Rinse the cauliflower and pat it dry. Remove the leaves and stem from the cauliflower, and then cut the head into small florets.
2. Use a food processor or blender to pulse the cauliflower florets until they reach the size of rice grains. If you don't have a food processor, you can grate the cauliflower with a box grater or chop it finely with a knife.
3. Heat the olive oil in a large skillet over medium-high heat. Add the diced onion and sauté it for 2-3 minutes or until it becomes translucent. Add the minced garlic and sauté for an additional minute, or until it becomes fragrant.
4. Add the diced carrot and frozen peas to the skillet and sauté for 3-4 minutes, or until the vegetables are tender.
5. Move the vegetables to one side of the skillet and pour the beaten eggs into the empty side. Scramble the eggs with a spatula until they are fully cooked, then combine them with the vegetables.
6. Introduce the riced cauliflower to the skillet and stir it in with the vegetables and eggs. Cook the mixture for 5-7 minutes or until the cauliflower becomes tender and turns light brown.
7. Pour soy sauce (or tamari or coconut aminos) into the skillet and stir it until the cauliflower is coated. Season with salt and black pepper to your liking.
8. Serve the fried cauliflower rice hot, garnished with sliced green onions, sesame seeds, and hot sauce if desired.

Per Serving
Calories: 121 | Fat: 5g |
Carbohydrates: 13g | Fiber: 4g | Sugar: 5g | Protein: 7g

Farley'S Muscle Building Chilli Con Carne

Prep time: 5 minutes | Cook time: 120 minutes | Serves 4

- 20oz lean ground beef
- 1 tbsp oil
- 1 chopped onion
- 1 chopped red pepper
- 2 crushed garlic cloves,
- 1 tsp of chilli powder
- 1 tsp paprika
- 1 tsp ground cumin
- 1 beef stock cube
- 16oz of tinned chopped tomatoes
- 2 tbsp tomato purée
- 16oz of dried and rinsed red kidney beans
- 1 cup of brown rice

Steps:

1. Get a pan and add the olive oil and heat on a medium heat.
2. Add the onions to the pan and fry until soft.
3. Then add the garlic, red pepper, chilli powder, paprika and cumin. Stir together and cook for 5 minutes.
4. Add the ground mince to the pan and cook until browned.
5. Get 300ml of hot water and add the beef stock cube to it. Add this to the pan along with the chopped tomatoes. Also add the puree and stir in well. Bring the pan to a simmer, cover and cook for around 50 minutes. Stir occasionally.
6. After 30 minutes and while the mince is cooking, add 300ml of cold water to a separate pot and heat until the water is boiling. Once boiling, add the rice and leave for 20 minutes.
7. Once the rice is done, drain and put to one side. Add the beans to the meat mix and cook for another 10 minutes.
8. Serve the rice topped with the chilli con carne.

Per Serving
Calories:389 | Protein: 37g | Carbs: 25g | Fat: 17g

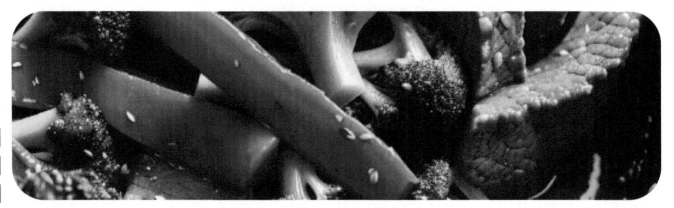

Chapter 13: Desserts

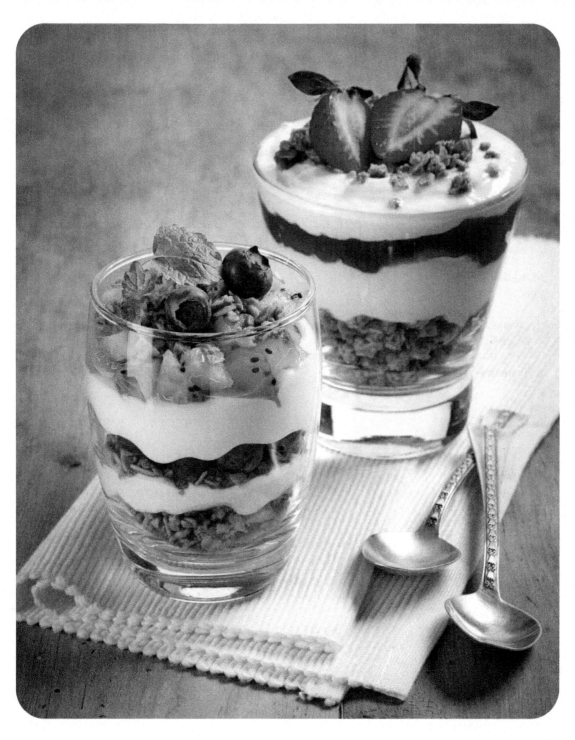

Turkey Apricot Roll-Ups

Prep time: 5 minutes | Cook time: 10 minutes | Serves 6

- 1 tablespoon apricot preserves
- 1 tablespoon dijon mustard
- 6 (1-ounce) slices deli roasted turkey

Steps:
1. Combine preserves and mustard in a small bowl. Mix well.
2. Spread turkey slices on a flat work space. Spoon about 1 teaspoon preserves mixture onto each slice of turkey and spread evenly. Roll turkey into cylinders. Serve immediately.

Per Serving

Calories: 26 | Fat: 0g | Sodium: 158mg | Carbohydrates: 3g | Fiber: 0g | Sugar: 2g | Protein: 3g

Ham and Swiss Rice Cakes

Prep time: 5 minutes | Cook time: 10 minutes | Serves 1

- 2 (.75-ounce) wedges creamy swiss spreadable cheese
- 2 plain salted rice cakes
- 2 teaspoons honey mustard
- 2 ounces sliced deli ham

Steps:
1. Spread one wedge of cheese on each rice cake. Top with honey mustard, then deli ham.
2. Serve immediately.

Per Serving

Calories: 210 | Fat: 9g | Sodium: 840mg | Carbohydrates: 19g | Fiber: 0g | Sugar: 4g | Protein: 14g

Protein Snack Box

Prep time: 5 minutes | Cook time: 10 minutes | Serves 1

- 3 ounces sliced deli turkey breast
- ½ large green bell pepper, seeded and sliced
- ½ cup cherry tomatoes
- 1 ounce cubed or sliced cheddar cheese
- 1 large hard-cooked egg

Steps:
1. Pile turkey slices in a stack and roll up to form a cylinder. Cut the cylinder crosswise into four pieces. Place turkey rolls in a glass storage container.
2. Arrange bell pepper slices, cherry tomatoes, cheese, and egg in the container. Cover and refrigerate for up to 3 days.

Per Serving

Calories: 289 | Fat: 15g | Sodium: 650mg | Carbohydrates: 9g | Fiber: 2g | Sugar: 7g | Protein: 30g

Peanut Butter Protein Cookies

Prep time: 5 minutes |Cook time: 15 minutes| Serves 10

- 1 cup natural peanut butter
- 2 large egg whites
- 1 scoop vanilla protein powder
- $^3/_4$ cup stevia
- 1 teaspoon cinnamon

Steps:
1. Preheat oven to 350°F.
2. Place all ingredients into a medium bowl and stir.
3. Shape dough into round cookies and spread out on a greased cookie sheet, leaving 1″ between cookies.
4. Bake 10 minutes, cool, and serve.

Per Serving (1 cookie):

Calories: 168 | Fat: 13 g | Protein: 8 g | Sodium: 95 mg | Fiber: 2 g | Carbohydrates: 8 g | Sugar: 3 g

Tuna Cucumber Bites

Prep time: 5 minutes | Cook time: 10 minutes | Serves 2

- 1 (5-ounce) can tuna, drained and flaked
- 1 tablespoon mayonnaise
- 1 tablespoon dijon mustard
- 1 medium cucumber, sliced into rounds

Steps:
1. Combine tuna, mayonnaise, and mustard in a small bowl. Mix together.
2. Place cucumber slices on a platter. Top each slice with a spoonful of the tuna mixture. Serve immediately.

Per Serving

Calories: 150 | Fat: 6g | Sodium: 457mg | Carbohydrates: 6g | Fiber: 1g | Sugar: 3g | Protein: 18g

Sweet Potato Baked Egg

Prep time: 5 minutes | Cook time: 10 minutes | Serves 1

- 1 medium sweet potato
- 1 teaspoon extra-virgin olive oil
- ⅛ teaspoon salt
- 2 large eggs

Per Serving

Calories: 317 | Fat: 17g | Sodium: 450mg | Carbohydrates: 24g | Fiber: 4g | Sugar: 7g | Protein: 16g

Steps:
1. Preheat oven to 425°F and line a baking sheet with parchment paper.
2. Slice sweet potato in half lengthwise and place cut side down on the prepared baking sheet. Brush with oil and sprinkle with salt. Bake for 30 minutes or until fork-tender.
3. Remove sweet potato halves from the oven and set aside to cool for 5–10 minutes until cool enough to handle. Use a spoon to scoop out some of the flesh from each half of the sweet potato to make room for the egg. Reserve scooped out sweet potato for another use.
4. Crack 1 egg into each hole and return sweet potato halves to the oven for 10–15 minutes. Bake for less time if you like your eggs runny, and bake longer if you like them firmer.
5. Remove from oven and serve immediately.

Peanut Butter Banana Frozen Greek Yogurt

Prep time: 5 minutes |Cook time: 5 minutes| Serves 1

- ½ cup Greek yogurt
- 1 medium frozen banana, sliced
- 2 tablespoons natural peanut butter

Steps:
Blend all ingredients in a blender or food processor until smooth and serve immediately.

Per Serving:

Calories: 362 | Fat: 16 g | Protein: 20 g | Sodium: 139 mg | Fiber: 5 g | Carbohydrates: 41 g | Sugar: 23 g

Roasted Carrot Bites

Prep time: 5 minutes | Cook time: 10 minutes | Serves 4

- 1 ½ pounds carrots, peeled and cut into ¼" slices
- 1 tablespoon olive oil
- ½ teaspoon salt

Steps:
1. Preheat oven to 425°F.
2. Combine carrots, oil, and salt in an oven-safe baking dish. Bake for 40–45 minutes, tossing carrots midway through cooking.
3. Turn off oven and leave carrots in the oven until they cool, about 90 minutes to 2 hours.
4. Remove from oven and serve immediately or refrigerate for up to 5 days.

Per Serving

Calories: 100 | Fat: 4g | Sodium: 288mg | Carbohydrates: 15g | Fiber: 5g | Sugar: 8g | Protein: 2g

High-Protein Oatmeal Cookies

Prep time: 5 minutes | Cook time: 15 minutes | Serves 12

- 1 $^3/_4$ cups dry oats
- 4 scoops vanilla protein powder
- $^1/_2$ cup applesauce
- $^1/_2$ cup egg whites
- 1 tablespoon olive oil
- 1 tablespoon stevia
- Dash cinnamon

Steps:
1. Preheat oven to 350°F.
2. Place ingredients in a large bowl and stir.
3. Shape dough into round cookies and spread out on a greased cookie sheet 1″ apart.
4. Bake 10–15 minutes, until lightly browned.

Per Serving (1 cookie):
Calories: 149 | Fat: 4 g | Protein: 9 g | Sodium: 46 mg | Fiber: 5 g | Carbohydrates: 21 g | Sugar: 2 g

Chocolate Banana Cups

Prep time: 5 minutes | Cook time: 10 minutes | Serves 8

- 1/2 cup chocolate chips
- 1/4 cup almond milk
- 1 medium banana, mashed

Per Serving
Calories: 88 | Fat: 4g | Protein: 1g | Sodium: 3mg | Fiber: 1g | Carbohydrates: 13g | Sugar: 9g

Steps:
1. In a small saucepan over medium-low heat, melt chocolate chips and almond milk together until soft.
2. Once melted, pour a small amount into the bottom of some lined mini-muffin cups, just enough to cover the bottom of the cups. This recipe should fill 8 mini cups, but may vary depending on the size you are using.
3. Place muffin tin in the freezer 5–10 minutes.
4. Remove muffin tin and add a bit of mashed banana to each cup.
5. Fill cups with remaining amount of chocolate, and return to freezer until ready to serve.

Protein Cheesecake

Prep time: 5 minutes | Cook time: 185 minutes | Serves 12

- 24 ounces fat-free cream cheese
- 2 scoops vanilla whey protein
- $^3/_4$ cup stevia
- 1 teaspoon vanilla extract
- 3 large eggs
- 1 tablespoon lemon juice

Steps:
1. Preheat oven to 350°F.
2. Place ingredients in a large bowl and mix with a hand mixer on medium speed.
3. Pour mix into a 9″ pie pan coated with nonstick cooking spray.
4. Bake 45 minutes and refrigerate 3 hours or until ready to serve.

Per Serving:
Calories: 177 | Fat: 3 g | Protein: 24 g | Sodium: 800 mg | Fiber: 0 g | Carbohydrates: 11 g | Sugar: 7 g

Lemon Coconut Protein Balls

Prep time: 5 minutes | Cook time: 10 minutes | Makes 12 balls

- ½ cup vanilla or coconut protein powder
- ½ cup melted coconut oil
- ¾ cup unsweetened shredded coconut
- 2 tablespoons honey
- 2 tablespoons lemon juice
- ½ teaspoon grated lemon zest
- 2 tablespoons coconut flour

Steps:
1. Line a large baking sheet with parchment paper.
2. Combine all ingredients in a large bowl. If the mixture is too crumbly, add water, 1 teaspoon at a time, until it holds together when squeezed.
3. Form the batter into 1″ balls and place on the prepared baking sheet. Refrigerate for at least 1 hour. Serve immediately or refrigerate for up to 1 week in a sealed container.

Per Serving
Calories: 185 | Fat: 15g | Sodium: 14mg | Carbohydrates: 7g | Fiber: 2g | Sugar: 3g | Protein: 5g

Appendix 1: Measurement Conversion Chart

MEASUREMENT CONVERSION CHART

VOLUME EQUIVALENTS(DRY)

US STANDARD	METRIC (APPROXIMATE)
1/8 teaspoon	0.5 mL
1/4 teaspoon	1 mL
1/2 teaspoon	2 mL
3/4 teaspoon	4 mL
1 teaspoon	5 mL
1 tablespoon	15 mL
1/4 cup	59 mL
1/2 cup	118 mL
3/4 cup	177 mL
1 cup	235 mL
2 cups	475 mL
3 cups	700 mL
4 cups	1 L

WEIGHT EQUIVALENTS

US STANDARD	METRIC (APPROXIMATE)
1 ounce	28 g
2 ounces	57 g
5 ounces	142 g
10 ounces	284 g
15 ounces	425 g
16 ounces (1 pound)	455 g
1.5 pounds	680 g
2 pounds	907 g

VOLUME EQUIVALENTS(LIQUID)

US STANDARD	US STANDARD (OUNCES)	METRIC (APPROXIMATE)
2 tablespoons	1 fl.oz.	30 mL
1/4 cup	2 fl.oz.	60 mL
1/2 cup	4 fl.oz.	120 mL
1 cup	8 fl.oz.	240 mL
1 1/2 cup	12 fl.oz.	355 mL
2 cups or 1 pint	16 fl.oz.	475 mL
4 cups or 1 quart	32 fl.oz.	1 L
1 gallon	128 fl.oz.	4 L

TEMPERATURES EQUIVALENTS

FAHRENHEIT(F)	CELSIUS(C) (APPROXIMATE)
225 °F	107 °C
250 °F	120 °C
275 °F	135 °C
300 °F	150 °C
325 °F	160 °C
350 °F	180 °C
375 °F	190 °C
400 °F	205 °C
425 °F	220 °C
450 °F	235 °C
475 °F	245 °C
500 °F	260 °C

Appendix 2: The Dirty Dozen and Clean Fifteen

The Dirty Dozen and Clean Fifteen

The Environmental Working Group (EWG) is a nonprofit, nonpartisan organization dedicated to protecting human health and the environment Its mission is to empower people to live healthier lives in a healthier environment. This organization publishes an annual list of the twelve kinds of produce, in sequence, that have the highest amount of pesticide residue-the Dirty Dozen-as well as a list of the fifteen kinds ofproduce that have the least amount of pesticide residue-the Clean Fifteen.

THE DIRTY DOZEN	THE CLEAN FIFTEEN
• The 2016 Dirty Dozen includes the following produce. These are considered among the year's most important produce to buy organic:	• The least critical to buy organically are the Clean Fifteen list. The following are on the 2016 list:

THE DIRTY DOZEN

- The 2016 Dirty Dozen includes the following produce. These are considered among the year's most important produce to buy organic:

Strawberries	Spinach
Apples	Tomatoes
Nectarines	Bell peppers
Peaches	Cherry tomatoes
Celery	Cucumbers
Grapes	Kale/collard greens
Cherries	Hot peppers

- *The Dirty Dozen list contains two additional itemskale/collard greens and hot peppers-because they tend to contain trace levels of highly hazardous pesticides.*

THE CLEAN FIFTEEN

- The least critical to buy organically are the Clean Fifteen list. The following are on the 2016 list:

Avocados	Papayas
Corn	Kiw
Pineapples	Eggplant
Cabbage	Honeydew
Sweet peas	Grapefruit
Onions	Cantaloupe
Asparagus	Cauliflower
Mangos	

- *Some of the sweet corn sold in the United States are made from genetically engineered (GE) seedstock. Buy organic varieties of these crops to avoid GE produce.*

Appendix 3: Index

Printed in Great Britain
by Amazon

47326639R00044